The Mother Elders

7 Laws of Feminine Power

Ann Lamb

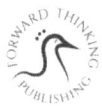

Forward Thinking Publishing

First published 2024

Published by Forward Thinking Publishing

Text © Ann Lamb (formerly Hobbs)

The moral rights of the author have been asserted.

All rights reserved. No part of this book may be reproduced by any mechanical, photographic or electronic process, or in the form of a phonographic recording; nor may it be stored in a retrieval system, transmitted or otherwise be copied for public or private use, other than for 'fair use' as brief quotations embodied in articles and reviews, without prior written permission of the publisher and author.

The information given in this book should not be treated as a substitute for professional medical advice; always consult a medical practitioner. Any use of information in this book is at the reader's discretion and risk. Neither the author nor the publisher can be held responsible for any loss, claim or damage arising out of the use, or misuse, of the suggestions made, the failure to take medical advice or for any material on third party websites.

A catalogue record for this book is available from the British Library.

ISBN: 978-1-916764-04-0

Published by Forward Thinking Publishing

Contents

CHAPTER 1 1

Introduction 1

What changes are you currently facing? 3

CHAPTER 2 8

What is Feminine Power? 8

Who are the Mother Elders? 11

What is the Mother Elders' definition of feminine power? 13

CHAPTER 3 15

7 Laws of Feminine Power 15

7 Laws of Feminine Power 18

CHAPTER 4 23

Law 1 – Harness Your Feminine Power 23

Meditation - Radiate your Feminine Power 33

CHAPTER 5 39

Law 2 – Build Loving Relationships 39

Being a Mother 41

Grieving our loss when children leave home 44

Relationship with Yourself 46

Relationships with Others 49

Dating Again 54

Seeking External Approval................................. 56

Coming back full circle – YOU 57

What do I want? 60

CHAPTER 6 61

Law 3 – Understand Your Power and Intuition ... 61

Your Ego 63

Trust 64

Ways in which we can listen............................... 67

Harness your words... 69

CHAPTER 7 71

Law 4 – Remain in Effortless Flow 71

Validation 72

How do we validate ourselves? 76

Have a powerful voice 78

Shine a light on your power 79

Meditation - Shine a light on your Soul 81

CHAPTER 8 85

Law 5 – Find Purpose in Life....................................85

How are you feeling right now? 86

It's not logical..88

It's not easy..89

Get clear on the next step 90

Allow yourself to flow...91

How to live a more fulfilling life 93

Meditation – Finding your Purpose 98

CHAPTER 9 104

Law 6 – Develop Your Spirituality.........................104

What stops us from building this spiritual connection?..111

Procrastination 112

What do you feel is your spiritual practice? 114

CHAPTER 10 116

Law 7 – Drop the Illusion 116

Who are you? 117

It's my fault 119

Who am I? 121

See yourself 123

Drop the illusion 124

Meditation – Uncovering the Real You 124

It's time to see yourself 128

CHAPTER 11 130

The Unspoken Law 130

Meditation - I am a Mother Elder 133

CHAPTER 12 138

How to Rise Collectively as Women 138

Loneliness 140

Community 142

What can you do? 142

CHAPTER 13 144

The Mother Elder **144**

About the Author..**147**

Where to find Ann **148**

Acknowledgments..**149**

"Each time a woman stands up for herself, without knowing it possibly, without claiming it, she stands up for all women."

– Maya Angelou

CHAPTER 1

Introduction

THE POWER OF THE feminine is sitting in your heart, an expression of love. I normally see the heart chakra as a red rose blossoming and opening, but in a recent coaching session, I came to see this expression of love as a powerful sun that radiated around my body.

It is not the heart chakra; it is something more powerful that we, as women, can direct, can use for good in the world, and can use to bring what we want into our own lives. This book is intended to teach you the seven laws of feminine power as told to me by my channel guides, the Mother Elders.

I am at a crossroads in my life where I have been a mother for the past 28 years and a wife for the last 30 or so years. This has been my identity for most of my life from the age of 19. I am now divorced, my children are all grown up and these events have led me to another chapter in my life. I have seen the parting of my children as painful, as a loss, and as something to grieve. I am no longer part of a family. I feel I no longer belong. I have no home. No identity as a mother or a woman.

I think these are natural feelings and ones that you may be feeling now. Some of you may have heard the expression 'empty nesters', but this brings in bad cognitions that something is missing, that we are in fact empty. This empty space allows our ego voice to be louder, the voice that tells us that no one loves us and that everyone has gone. We feel lost and unsure of our footing. Some of you reading this book may be thinking, "Have I still got a purpose in life?" I know I am.

However, if we see this passing as a transition into another chapter of our lives then we let go of the ego's ability to keep us small, to tell us that we are not good enough. It is interesting that, at the same time as my children are leaving, my body is transitioning from producing babies to being in menopause. There are so many changes that are occurring in this stage of our lives; our bodies, our outer lives and our relationships are changing. No wonder we don't feel balanced, that we feel we are on uneven ground. Are you feeling like this? Take a moment to pause and consider this.

What changes are you currently facing?

It is only when we bring awareness to this question that we can start to heal. I know I have avoided this question for a long time by keeping busy and by losing myself in work. It is time, as women, to consider these changes. We owe it to ourselves and more importantly, teach other women who may be facing these challenges. When you change, other women are watching and this is important to be aware of. You are not only changing for yourself but for other women too.

We keep busy because our ego doesn't want us to pause long enough to ask this question. It wants us to fight these feelings, to be angry at our bodies because we are no longer menstruating and unable to bear children. It tells us that we are 'past our sell-by date' and that we no longer have a purpose as a woman.

What if, and I put this concept to you so that you can meditate on it and come to your own conclusions, we celebrate this passing as one of our feminine powers? That this phase of our lives is calling us to truly be powerful and stand in our feminine power. How powerful that we, as women, go through this transition in our lives and still our femininity burns freely and more powerfully than ever before. That we have now transitioned into this period of our lives where we have more wisdom than ever before. What a concept!

One day when on a walk out in nature, I heard a voice (not sure where it was coming from) and I was asked a question. I was being asked if I would allow these guides, the Mother Elders, to teach me the laws of feminine power. All I heard was, "Are you ready to receive this information?" As I was relaxed and contented, I said yes, curious as I never believed in these guides before. My spiritual friend said I must have been in the right place to receive this information and that before then I would have totally freaked out. I believe in healing, and when I work I sometimes feel the presence of my sister in spirit, but I had never believed in anything else, until now.

I am not sure whether it is my own voice or my own wisdom that I am sharing but nevertheless, I have felt that everything that has come through me has helped me to transition through this period of my life.

To be truthful I said yes, thinking that they would guide me out of the pain that I was feeling over the loss of my children, to help me find the answer to where my home was. However, something bigger came into being. The guides said that they would give me the '7

Laws of Feminine Power' and that I must translate that into what it means in the western world. Whether you believe that or not, you don't have to, even I don't know why these Mother Elders chose me to put this out into the world. I was curious enough at first to explore how I could use these laws in my own life so that I could understand the meaning in order to teach other people. All the books that I write come from my own experiences, and what I have transformed in my life, so I suppose this book is no different.

Over the last few years, the world has seen these strange times of being in lockdown with COVID-19, and during that period we paused for those two years. Nowhere to go, no distractions of being busy; we had simply had more time to reflect. Even now things have not gone back to what they had been.

There are many of us, particularly women, who will rise and be awakened by having had some downtime, this time of pause that the whole world experienced together. It is in these periods of downtime that we will be able to listen more clearly to our feminine powers and our intuition. These are the times when literally the world had stopped where we can no longer go out and fill those spaces that we have in the past with busyness, work, and family. We are forced to sit with ourselves and maybe conclude that we are no longer happy with where we are.

In this period, we have seen how our work changed: people are no longer happy going into the office five days a week; they prefer to have more time at home. People are valuing their freedom rather than the 9–5 hamster wheel that we have all been on for many years.

Perhaps you are seeking more in your life, realising that your relationships are no longer working and, like me, finding yourself on your own. I have family and my children, but they no longer need me in the context of how I have been serving them for the past 30 years. Now you may say that that's exciting, I can start a new life but it doesn't feel as simple as that. My friends have told me that I have done a good job of parenting my children as they are now independent young men, but that doesn't help with the feelings of loss and thoughts of, "What the f*** am I going to do now with my life?"

If you are in a similar position to me then this book will help you transition to becoming the Mother Elder, to have a purpose to your life, and to start living the life you want. The life you deserve without the distraction of what we 'should' be doing or what other people think we 'ought' to be doing.

If you are one of these women then come along with me on this journey.

CHAPTER 2

What is Feminine Power?

I'M NOT SURE WHY I received this message about femininity because I feel I have denied mine from an early age. In school I was always tall but I wanted to be short. I never wanted to stand out so I denied my own identity and tried to fit in. I feel I have also abused this femininity by losing myself in relationships and have been frightened of my femininity. But what is femininity? How is it defined?

The definition in the Oxford Dictionary says:

Femininity: qualities or attributes regarded as characteristic of women.

Feminine: having qualities or an appearance traditionally associated with women.

These are what I would call stereotypical and surface layers of being a woman.

What does power mean?

Power: the ability or capacity to do something or act in a particular way.

Both male and female have both feminine and masculine qualities but I feel women have stronger feminine qualities. If women live too much in their masculinity, then it will lead to burn-out. However, over the years I have felt women are seen as the weaker sex because we have more feminine qualities. What do you think?

Now let's look at my definition of feminine power.

My definition of feminine power is the beauty within us all, whether man or woman. It is our intuition based on feelings and emotions. We instinctively know what is right or wrong and we can listen to our higher power.

That is what feminine power is about. How would you define your feminine power?

However, as I said in the introduction, we are taught to use it in a different way. When we start using it in a positive way our lives become better, we begin to live our more powerful selves. We are more content and happier.

You may be thinking feminine power is the spiritual part of us, and if you are not spiritual then you cannot access it. I don't believe that is true. If we embrace our feminine power, then we begin to uncover the truth of who we are.

When I was a life coach, people came to me to be 'fixed' as they believed that something was wrong with them. However, on my own journey of self-development and helping many other people, I believe that what we do during the journey of self-discovery is uncovering our true self. We become at one with ourselves. There is nothing wrong, we don't need to fix anything as we are not broken. We have just been conditioned and that is what we need to explore and remove, the conditioning and not our true personality. We just need to uncover and get back to the core of who we are to live our lives to the fullest.

I believe over the years women have been told that their femininity is a weakness. I have been told on many occasions that I am too emotional, and this has led me to become harder, to be more masculine in my life.

However, this is not what our feminine power is about.

This feminine power is what will help us in our lives if we use it right.

Who are the Mother Elders?

As I said in the introduction, the Mother Elders came through me when I was walking in the fields. They asked if I wanted the wisdom that they needed to share and I said yes. I believe they have come through me to help me in my own life. It is fascinating that every chapter that I have written I have either gone through or transitioned into after writing the chapter. One time I asked a very good friend a question which she answered. A couple of days later I was re-writing this book and I looked at a particular paragraph. It was exactly what my friend had said to me. I couldn't believe that I had written it several months before. That is the power of this book and the information that I share within it.

When I connect to the Mother Elders, I envision them as a group of women sitting in a circle around a fire. There is an elder Mother Elder who stands guard. I envision her as a long-haired grey woman standing by the fire. She invites me into the circle. I then see all the other Mother Elders. They each have their place. When I envision them in my mind's eye, I am calm, I feel at peace, and feel that I am being nurtured. There is no judgement. I can go and sit and share my problems. These are the Mother Elders.

As I write this book, I believe we are all Mother Elders, especially when we go through menopause, whether in the early stages (perimenopausal) or right through to when our periods stop (menopause). In this period, I believe that this is the most powerful time that we are in our feminine power. We have gone through life, raised children, or not, led a fulfilling life and we have so much wisdom to share. These are what the Mother Elders are sharing with us: their wisdom. When women go into menopause some might call us 'old crones'. I do not like the word 'old crone' as to me, this is not a true representation of where I am in my life. I like to think of it as I have simply grown into a wise woman. What do you think?

Over the years I have enjoyed sharing my wisdom when teaching others about self-development and now as a publisher. Sharing our wisdom and what we are going through or have been through helps so many people. I remember sharing that I had panic attacks in my 20s and the response I got back was, 'so did I'. I didn't realise it was common. I felt I was the only one experiencing them. After I heard that, a huge weight was lifted off my shoulders and I began to feel better and felt that I wasn't failing at life. However, we do fail to share what is going on in our lives and even menopause is a hush-hush topic. However, I believe if we share our wisdom then it will help other people like it did me. We begin to see that what we are experiencing is common and, in that, we don't feel so alone. Even when your friends ask you, "How are you?" it is crucial that you are truthful. If we politely say everything is okay, they might think that they are the only ones feeling this way. Even when I speak about my perimenopausal symptoms, it is a huge relief when my friends say, "Oh yes, I had this."

I hope that you will begin to see that our feminine power is to nurture and be patient with ourselves as we transition into a Mother Elder.

What is the Mother Elders' definition of feminine power?

When I asked this question of the Mother Elders, this was their response:

We see this feminine power that you talk about as an inner radiance that all beings have. Women are more in tune with this than men, but we all have this inner radiance. It is a natural state, a natural being that you humans have forgotten. You are too busy in the doing that you forget to use the natural being. When you do nothing and forget everything, this natural being is strong. That is what you are tapping into, this natural force. That is why we are bringing you the seven laws of feminine power; because we believe that you need this information. You need to remember how to be in relationships, in the world, and how to reconnect with your feminine power. It is in everyone. But you have forgotten. We are here to bring you this information so that you can remember the power of the feminine natural force.

In the next chapter, we focus on what the seven laws of feminine power are, so as the Mother Elders say, we can reconnect to this feminine power.

CHAPTER 3

7 Laws of Feminine Power

I BELIEVE WE HAVE been using our feminine power wrongly for many years. It may be due to violence against women and abusive relationships, but also the assumption that women get what they want by using their sexual powers to manipulate others. Sometimes this hasn't been in real life, but we see so many of these scenarios play out in films and the like.

You may be wondering if feminine power is the same as sexuality. I believe they are all the same as we are one. We are not separate from our powers or our emotions, but what is true is that we have not used these powers for the greater good.

The definition to me of the word 'power' frightens me a little. I don't want to control others. I don't want to be manipulative. Therefore, how can we reframe the word 'power' to mean something positive? Like the quote from the Mother Elders said in the previous chapter, this 'power' is a natural force, it is within all of us.

The power can mean that we must control our own lives to create how we want our lives to be and to manifest the things and relationships that enrich and nourish our bodies. When I was a life coach, I coached many people, and the one thing I noticed and said to my clients regularly was, "You can't change anybody or anything else other than yourself." With that phrase in mind, therefore, the power you have in your feminine body cannot do anybody other than you harm. Whether we use this power negatively or positively, this power is for your use only.

I know I have used my power more in a negative way. When I moan about things, I get a headache. When I worry and overthink, I feel tired. These are all still uses of our power. However, when I do use it in a way that enriches my life, I feel uplifted and happy. I don't overthink, I just do. I am happy and fulfilled. How has this played out in your life? Make a list of how you have used this power negatively and positively within yourself and you will begin to see a pattern in your life. Do you want to change that? Do you want to transition into a woman who uses her feminine power for the greater good?

If the answer is yes, then you are in the right place, and we will go together on this journey to explore what this feminine power is all about, how we can use it in our lives, and how we can share it with others. I am, by no means, there yet. I don't think I ever will be, but I am open to the learnings and the possibility that, though I am no longer a mother and a bearer of children, I am still of value. I am indeed a Mother Elder, and if you are reading this then you are too.

We will explore these seven laws of feminine power together and see where they can be applied in our lives. I will decipher and interpret them based on what has been happening in my life and how I want my life to move forward. I am a powerful human being. I know that deep down I have manifested great things in my life. I work with wonderful authors, and I have a beautiful family and wonderful friends, but it is now time for me to explore, not necessarily who I am without my role as a mother, but rather, how I can begin this new chapter in my life.

These are the seven laws that I will write in more detail about in the following chapters as told to me by the Mother Elders. Please read these laws and start thinking about what they mean to you. Use your feminine power to pause and consider what each law means to you. Perhaps they might mean different things to you than me or to the next woman that you share this book with, and that is okay. Life has different meanings to us all but know that you are being guided to be your own guru. I am simply planting a seed so that you can fully blossom. I give you permission to use your feminine power to enrich and nourish your soul.

7 Laws of Feminine Power

Law 1 - Harness your feminine power - What is your feminine power and how do you see it? In essence, this is how you see yourself. Take a look in the mirror to find your glow, to find your superpowers that lie within your feminine body. You can do this by taking care of yourself, dressing well, eating well, and knowing and having faith that this feminine power will help you in your life. See yourself as a woman in power and how you would use this power. It must be used for the greater good of all.

Law 2 – Build loving relationships – Look at your relationship with yourself and with others.

Do these people ignite your power or diminish it? Do you give away your feminine power willingly to make others accept you and love you? Really look at these external relationships and how they are serving you. Heal the linear line so that these patterns and mistakes do not happen again. Review where you have been with relationships and where you would like to go to harness your feminine power. For some being a mother is one of the highest orders that a woman is being called for. Although we feel abandoned by our children when they grow up, it is time to understand our role in parenting these young children and what our duties are as mothers. We shape the future.

Law 3 – Understand your power and intuition
- Feminine power remains in all of us, men or women although women are more in tune with it. However, women do not understand their own capabilities and let the ego talk them out of it. They do not listen to their own intuition and seek help from others. They need to learn to listen to themselves whether they are spiritual or not.

Law 4 – Remain in effortless flow - Relationships can be the feminine power's downfall. You lose yourself and begin to move away from who you are. You are being called to stay within that power and to ground your femininity. Many of you in the western world do not understand what femininity is. You understand it as a curse and not a blessing. However, if women understand their power and remain open to all aspects of love. They will advance you to the next level and will teach you many things.

Seek approval only from yourself. Do not look at others to make you happy or to make you feel complete. Seek approval from your inner being and your guides. Meditate and sit quietly and listen to your intuition and tune into your guides. Your guides are always around you, so use this inner GPS. Seek approval from only yourself.

Law 5 – Find purpose in life - Everyone is looking for purpose in life, in what you do in a job. When things fall away, when kids leave home, you are still looking for a purpose in life. However, your purpose on this earth is to just be you. The difficulty is that you can lose yourself in relationships, in being a mother, and then you are surprised when you have no purpose. This is not true for us, the Mother Elders. Our purpose is to be here, to be ourselves, and to brighten each other's day. It is not all about doing stuff and pushing and pulling. It's about knowing that the purpose of your life is to be happy and stop doing. Just be.

Law 6 - Develop your spirituality – Develop a practice to help you to develop your spirituality. Procrastination stops the flow and you cannot develop your spirituality. Make it a priority in your life. When you procrastinate, you dampen your energetic flow and become blinded. You cannot see anything. The Mother Elders do not understand why you would procrastinate if you don't have time to do the things you want to do. Make time and make sure they are important enough for you to stick to the regime. Notice your inner critic.

Law 7 – Drop the illusion - Be you. There is no one else like you out there in the world. You are always trying to find out who you are. How many times have we heard prayers of "please tell me who I am" as if this is a mystery to all human beings? There is no path to finding yourself. This is just an illusion. The illusion is that you don't *see* who you are. You think you know who you are, but it's a false sense of self. See yourself in the mirror. Drop the ego and the illusion of who you *think* you are. See who you are with a new set of eyes. The set of eyes that we, the Mother Elders, see. We see you with our hearts. It is time to see yourself in this way too.

When you read these laws, what has come up for you? Always go with your first instinct don't analyse and overthink what is coming into your intuition. Find a quiet space and journal to reflect on what they mean. As I said, they might mean different things to you, and that is okay.

- What law most resonates with you at this time as you read them?

Don't overthink. Go with the first thing that comes into your mind.

How you use these laws is up to you, but I know from my experience that I have used these to the detriment of myself, more negatively than positively. Isn't it about time that we use the feminine laws more positively?

Let's journey together to explore how we have used them to our detriment and how we can begin to learn to use these more positively to create the next chapter in our lives. We will start with how to harness your feminine power.

CHAPTER 4

Law 1 - Harness Your Feminine Power

"See yourself as a woman in power and how you would use this power."

IF I ASKED YOU, "What is your feminine power and how do you see it?" What would you answer?

Take time to reflect on the following questions:

- Do you see this power as something that you don't have?

- Are you unsure of how to access your feminine power?

As I mentioned in Chapter 1, some feminine powers are stereotypically part of the feminine being and they might be traits such as nurture, sensitivity, sweetness, supportiveness, gentleness, warmth, cooperativeness, expressiveness, modesty, humility, empathy, affection, tenderness, emotional, kind, helpful, and devoted.

When you read these traits what do you feel? Have you been told that these traits are weak? I know that I am an emotional feminine being and have been told on numerous occasions that I'm "over-emotional," and I "cry all the time." Do you resonate with this? What have you been told throughout your life?

To harness your feminine power, you must look at yourself and, in essence, understand what feminine power means to you and how you see yourself. Not one fits all as we are all individuals. You must see yourself totally naked (not literally) but free from the limitations that life has placed upon you. Look in the mirror to find your glow, to find your superpowers that lie within your feminine body. Sometimes you might not be able to put words to your superpowers. You may only feel what it means. See how it feels to stand in this power. Practice how it feels to stand solid in your feminine power.

What do you see? How do you feel?

By beginning to understand yourself on a deeper level this will help you with your connection to life and your relationship with others. As I said in *Kick Ass Your Life* (my first book), shining a light on yourself is the first step to transformation and, in this context, it is the first step to regaining and harnessing your feminine power.

See the traits that you discern in yourself as your superpowers and that harnessing them will bring you what you want in your life. Rather than bringing negative connotations to them and placing limitations upon what you don't see as brilliant, bring these words to life by thinking positively about your feminine powers.

Even if you see some flaws in what you see like 'I'm too emotional,' just accept them. They are a part of you and by denying this, you deny all your feminine powers. If you perceive them as wrong then you are falling into the limitations that people have placed upon you all your life. Don't make them wrong, drop the conditioning that has been placed on you, be proud of them, and make them something that makes you an individual, stand tall and be proud. Acceptance is key to transformation.

For example, to be a great mother you need all those traits to nurture and protect your children. So, you might be able to see what your superpowers are, but you may be struggling, like me, to find how you can use these traits in your life now without children. The finite answer is to use these feminine traits on yourself. Nurture yourself. Does even that suggestion feel weird?

When someone says nurture someone else, I'm there, doing things naturally. However, if someone says to nurture myself, I go into a tailspin and have no idea how to do that. That's fine, we just haven't been taught how to do that. Society tells us that we are selfish in thinking about ourselves, about putting ourselves first as we are told family always comes first. Sit for one minute and consider how your life will look if you nurture YOU.

How would that feel?

What would you do to nurture yourself?

Sometimes we look outside of ourselves when we want to feel nurtured. I remember going to see a therapist when my marriage first broke up and all I wanted her to do was nurture me and fill me back up. I had no idea how to do that for myself. Over the years I've known, most of the time, what I've needed. It has been a process, but the funny thing is that I have always known what I needed but I just thought it was wrong. When I get too emotional, I like to get out of the house. I've dealt with this by thinking I'm running away and that I must sit with the emotion. However, when my body is pulsating with emotions, the best thing for me is to go out in nature and take a walk. In no way does it suggest that I'm running away from my emotions. I will deal with them but not when they are so heightened. Over the years I have compared myself with others and how they deal with things. We are all different so there is no right or wrong.

What takes me out of my feminine power is to beat myself up about it, by not acknowledging that nurturing myself means that I need to take a walk. By nurturing myself I need to be gentle with myself, to love myself even more. We just haven't been taught, as women, how to do that.

I invite you to take some time to get to know what it means to you to take care of yourself. Does it mean that you wear clothes that make you feel good about yourself? Or, by eating better, filling your body with nourishing foods? Sit with this for a moment and see what words or pictures jump into your mind. Write them down and journal about them. Don't make them wrong or compare them with others. This is unique to you and one size doesn't fit all. It is up to you to use your feminine power to find out your own answers.

Have faith that your feminine power will help you in your life, it is indeed a strength if you learn to harness the feminine power. See yourself as a woman in her feminine power, you are an individual and will have individual qualities. Don't compare yourself with others and your friends. We are not the same. You are an individual so celebrate that fact. Love yourself unconditionally.

When you recognise your feminine powers, these are also your superpowers, your strengths. This is where you need self-awareness to really dig deep, and to know your strengths. You might think that some of these feminine powers are a weakness but if you learn how to harness everything about yourself then they will become your strength. As I said before being emotional is not a weakness, it is a strength. Being sensitive is a strength but also can be perceived as a weakness. By getting to know what your superpowers are you learn how to work with them all. It may feel vulnerable at first but vulnerability is a great gift to have. We simply have not been taught how to harness all our gifts.

We all have different strengths which builds our unique personality. In the twenty-first century, women have so many choices, but the Mother Elders have told me:

We, Mother Elders, had no problems because we were not stripped of our feminine power, we knew our place and our power and this was not stripped. The western world strips you of this power, we are unsure why, but probably because they do not see your feminine power because you have not been taught to harness it within yourselves.

I'm not sure how you relate to this, but my view is that we live in a masculine world, corporate life is structured for men, and I have seen many clients who do not fit into this masculine world. I know I have burnt out many times trying to keep up with these structures.

They clearly do not fit us as women and certainly do not cater to women who menstruate or stop menstruating. We are also trying to be too many things: a mother, a career woman, etc. We can be all these things if we learn to harness our feminine power. That means we can't work like men. We need nourishment at certain times of our lives and these structures in the twenty-first century don't suit us. That is why it is up to us as women to make a stand and we cannot do this if we deny our feminine power, to make it wrong. That is why is it important that you look at harnessing this power.

You can practice this by firstly accepting who you are and where you are right now. Firstly, accept where you are. Don't beat yourself up or apologise as this is a good starting point. The first step to any change is awareness and acceptance. Become aware of where you are right now and accept it. You didn't know any better and you are reading this book for more information.

Secondly, you need to honour this feminine power. Try not to become overwhelmed with masculinity, the *doing*, femininity is about *being*. To be, you need to sit in prayer/meditation or sit with yourself. It is as powerful as *doing* something. This is where we have missed out in the western world because we are continually doing, doing, and doing. We are not simply *being*. There is no time to just sit and be.

During the period of COVID, many people were forced to stop and to pause. Some people would have accepted this and sat with themselves. Many would have got themselves in a state of depression and felt isolated with their thoughts. We have lost the art of just being. The Mother Elders have told me that in the western world, we do not sit in community with other women anymore. They also explained that:

You don't sit in a circle when menstruation happens like we have done as Mother Elders. You are overlooked and you must carry on like normal. In menstruation you need this space, this allowance to just be a woman and this is denied you in the western world. Just to be a woman. What does that feel like for you in the western world? There is no separation between women and men. You have to be all one person and be torn into two. This is not your feminine power, you have forgotten what it is, what it feels like, and how to harness it.

How do you feel about what the Mother Elders say? Do you agree or not? How do we celebrate menstruation, PMT and menopause? I know I grew up not talking and communicating about what was going on. We were told to keep it secret and that it was 'women's problems.' That may have changed but not in my generation. At menopause we are told that we are getting older, no longer can bear children and are therefore useless. No one says that we are, in fact, getting wiser.

Society seems to disregard women and the changes and flows that women have to deal with. Some of this is changing as I write this book with companies making concessions for women in menopause. But will this alienate women and men and be seen as a weakness in the workplace? Is society telling us that we need to keep up with men and if we do not then we are the weaker sex? We need to celebrate that we are different without causing separation. Men and women have different needs and therefore work in different ways. This can be celebrated.

The Mother Elders also say:

You begin to do this by honouring yourself as a woman. You have brought life into this world, you have nurtured your children selflessly not thinking about yourself and therefore you have forgotten that you are a woman, your needs haven't been met. So now you have time in menopause to give back to yourself, you have forgotten what to do. We need to remind you. To sit in community. To sit with yourself and just be. *Sit in the sunshine, sit in quietness and stillness without an agenda.*

So, for today, sit in stillness outside. Just walk with no thoughts in your mind. Empty your head and just walk. Take off your shoes and connect with the earth. Walk and just *be*. Feel in your body what that feels like, don't judge but just see how this feels. It will feel weird and uncomfortable at first, but the more you do this the more you connect with your body. Feel the sensations in your body. Do not try and analyse; just see them as floating in and out, like your thoughts in meditation. A feeling is just a feeling, it floats in and out.

By harnessing this feminine power, it is to come back to these powers, to fully embody them everywhere in your body. Give life back to yourself. Give yourself space to be fully present without an agenda. This is the first step in coming back to yourself and harnessing your feminine power.

This meditation will help you to enter that state of *being*.

Meditation - Radiate your Feminine Power

Find a quiet place where you can sit. Or, go out for a walk, be outside in nature, or sit on the grass. Anywhere you like, just for the connection, whatever feels good for you. Take a couple of deep breaths and close your eyes if you wish.

Breathe in.

Breathe out.

When you breathe out release everything that is not serving you right now. It can be emotions or tension in your body - anything that you are holding on to.

Breathe in, breathe out.

On the out breath release all the expectations that you have placed upon yourself, all the 'should's' and the 'must's'. Does it feel heavy? Where are you feeling this heaviness?

Do you feel in your power? Or do you feel powerless?

What do these words mean in your body? How are you feeling them? How are you receiving them?

Breathe in, breathe out.

Imagine a bright yellow sun in your heart. You can direct this sun wherever you like. You can radiant this sun out into all aspects of your body, to heal where you are hurting, to heal your thoughts. To heal your body. To heal your scars.

Firstly, radiate this bright yellow sun out from the heart, shooting bits off all over the body, move this feeling and radiate this sun all around your body. Soak yourself in this feeling, bask in this yellow sun.

Sit or walk and bask in this brilliant sunshine. It is hot, it nourishes your body. It nurtures your womb. It nurtures your whole being. Just sit for a while whilst this sun gets hotter and hotter.

Breathe in and breathe out.

Feel these words in your body as I speak them.

You are wonderful.

You are a powerful feminine woman.

You are amazing.

Then say to yourself, I forgive myself.

I allow myself to express myself fully.

I give myself permission to stand proud in my feminine power.

Let this power of the sun give you permission. The Universe gives you this permission if you don't fully trust yourself to give yourself this.

You may not understand or be aware of this feminine power yet, but it is there, deep inside of you and as we move along this journey you will feel it more present in you. You will be able to direct this sun, this feminine power, to all areas of your life.

Radiate this brilliant sunshine where you harness the feminine power. Do you accept this strong feminine power? Start right now and honour where you have been, and where you are going in this present moment. Honour yourself.

You have done a good job as a mother, a wife, a daughter, and a sister. There is no loss, only new life. You are a wise wisdom now as you transition through your life.

Breathe in, breathe out.

Create an image in your mind's eye of this wise woman. She is standing in her feminine power in front of you. What do you see?

What does she look like?

Are you able to connect with her?

Can you see her clearly or is she faded?

No matter what, feel her, feel the wise woman emerging from your being. Harness this power, harness this wise woman.

Give her a name. Call her into being if this makes it more real.

The Mother Elders are here to guide you through the next journey of your womanhood, into this wise woman.

They say, we are calling you back to your feminine power. You have been lost and we are brought here to guide you back to yourself.

Call upon your own wise woman to give you a message. Sit quietly for a few minutes as you receive this wonderful message.

Do not try and analyse this message. Lift your hands to receive this and then say thank you.

Honour this voice, this is in your inner knowing, your wise woman. Sit with your hands folded in prayer as you feel this presence and honour yourself.

Breathe in, breathe out.

When you are ready lets this image float away, wriggle your fingers and toes and come back to the present moment.

Take time to journal what you felt, saw or heard. It will help to remind yourself of the message that you were given. Don't worry if you have forgotten or didn't get a message. It is more important to ask these questions and let the answers come to you. The answers may take time to follow. Know that everything is working out perfectly, you are in the perfect moment, taking time for yourself. That is far more important. You can do this meditation again anytime you feel like you have lost the connection with your wise woman.

When travelling last year in France I felt my own wise woman. I was walking on a beach and suddenly I was standing taller, I felt my hair blowing in the wind, I felt strong. I felt free. There were no thoughts of 'I'm not good enough,' no thoughts at all. I want you to feel this connection to your own wise woman because when I hit a brick wall I imagine and feel this wise woman. It brings me strength and joy.

I want to share my experiences with you to return you to this wise woman. The Mother Elders are helping us all to return to our own inner wisdom and feminine power.

CHAPTER 5

Law 2 - Build Loving Relationships

"Heal the linear line so that you can heal your patterns."

LOVING RELATIONSHIPS ARE NOT always about loving other people. If you are a mother, like me, then you will know that most of our love is poured into our children. You have done a great job of bringing up your children. The Mother Elders tell me that being a mother is one of the highest orders that a woman is being called to. If you think about all the traits of being a feminine woman, as set out in Chapter 2, we use our feminine power for the greatest good when we are mothers. We are nurturing, loving, kind, supportive, gentle and empathic, and give unconditional love to our children. These qualities are our feminine power.

We must nurture relationships as they are not easy, and that is why so many marriages fail when the children leave. I know I was one of them. When my children started to leave, I realised that I had nothing in common with my ex-husband. We had done the classic pouring everything into our children and forgetting about our relationship as husband and wife.

On the other hand, relationships, and their failure gives us useful messages that we can use elsewhere in our lives. They also give us an indication of whether we give our feminine power away when we are in relationships.

This law reminds us to remain open to all aspects of love whether they serve us in the way we want them to. When we think we are in the wrong relationship or being tested by our children, these lessons, the Mother Elders remind us, will advance us to the next level and will teach us many things.

There are many kinds of relationships we will encounter during our lives. Some of which are positive and others that seem to be negative. However, the Mother Elders inform us that all relationships hold a message for us. Let's look at the different relationships that we may have already encountered in our lives.

Being a Mother

In this Law, the Mother Elders say:

> *Being a mother is one of the highest orders that women are being called to.*

I felt abandoned when my children started to leave home. My friends advised me to look at the situation in a different way in that I've done a good job as a mother. I nurtured them and gave them skills to be independent. I have shaped their futures. How powerful is that? That is why the Mother Elders remind us that being a mother is one of the highest orders. I hope you feel that way too.

Being a mother is a powerful thing and one, I feel, that shapes the future of our next generation. This is such a powerful way to look at it. What an amazing job we are doing to prepare the next generation for greatness. It is a tough job, we don't always get it right and there were many times that I told my children, "You didn't come with a manual." I certainly didn't get it right all the time but when I look at my children now, they seem to be independent and well-grounded young men.

Our duty as mothers has also shaped *us*. It has allowed us to express our feminine power to an extent that it comes naturally but, nevertheless, we must acknowledge it as our feminine power. Don't forget what we said in the introduction about power, it isn't to rule over people or to get what we want, it is a power that comes naturally to us when we look after other people. We harness it well within the relationship of being a mother. However, we do not use that same feminine power on ourselves or use it to its fullest potential in other situations. Why do you think that is?

Deep down I know I've done a great job, sometimes I think maybe too great of a job as my children are now all independent. They no longer need me on a day-to-day basis, but the truest comfort is that I know I will be the first person they call if they are in trouble or want some advice. I have three boys, now in their twenties. One of my sons lived in Canada for a year or so. When I thought he no longer needed me, I had a call and he said, "I'm not happy." I went into 'mother mode' and said, "Come home, life is too short to be unhappy." I felt needed again. I could be there for him, give him advice, and show him how much love I had to give to him.

You may feel that when your children are leaving home you haven't done a great job. I have felt grief and loss every time one of my children has left. At the time I couldn't understand why I was feeling like this and I listened to others telling me that these feelings were wrong. The first time my son went off to University, I felt that I had abandoned him and I still have that same feeling that they have abandoned me because they are leaving. You may also have the feeling that they don't care and that is why they are leaving. That's fine, they are just emotions that you need to express and to accept the way you are feeling. Sometimes it is not a logical feeling at all.

When I was in the midst of grief somebody said to me, "See your children as an arrow and you are the bow. You are just shooting them out into the world." That story did make me feel better, but I still had a sense of loss within me that lasted a few years. (I am still trying to figure out that feeling).

If you have been a mother, you are indeed a very strong and loving person, you can't not be.

Your children will bring the best and worst out in you. Do you ever think that they have picked up one of your bad traits and feel guilty? I have on many occasions but, writing this book, I think I have failed to see the 'good' traits.

My other son is in a relationship and I look at him as he is very loving and caring and does everything for his girlfriend. His relationship with me has also changed and he is very protective of me now. Where did he learn those traits? Well, you might ask yourself that, some has come from my parenting and being a loving mum and I'm proud of that. What are you proud of?

Grieving our loss when children leave home

It is logical to think that our children will grow up and leave but our emotions will think otherwise. I believe this is a natural process to grieve when your children leave home. You have nurtured them for over 20 years and you feel a sense of responsibility for them. Maybe we are also grieving for ourselves, that we have lost our identity as a mother. However, when I started to grieve when my children left home other people would make comments like; you know your kids will leave home! They made me feel wrong about my emotions and I had many people ask me, "Why are you so sad?" And when my son left, he said, "Why is she so upset? I'm not dying."

Grief is a funny emotion and one that I feel women need to express. If we do not then it stagnates in our bodies and becomes an issue in the future. Grieving is a natural process and one that may bring up other losses in our lives. Don't forget it is just a feeling. When my youngest son left home, I couldn't bear to sit in the family home and be on my own, so it prompted me to sell up, leave home and go travelling.

I thought this was so I didn't need to sit in my grief and pain, but you always bring that pain with you so it doesn't work. However, what I think I needed to do was to find a way to express my grief, to move on without my children. It is hard even now to think about losing my children but as an 'empty nester' it is just another path that I am on. I am on the path of self-discovery that will lead me to the next chapter of my life.

When I don't have the distraction of caring for my children or loving a partner, it leaves a void, a space. I believe that space is for me to explore myself, and to have a deeper relationship with myself that I have been avoiding over the years.

It feels strange that it is only me, I am indeed on my own. It also forces me to look closely at myself, to have a relationship with ME.

Relationship with Yourself

You may be thinking 'why is it vital to be in a relationship with myself?' You are the most important person in the world to you, and thus it's beneficial to be kind to yourself, nurture yourself, and grow - all the things you give to your children as a parent. We have already established that you are a great mother and you have written down what you are most proud of. Do you extend those proud moments to yourself?

Although I have been teaching self-development for many years, I still find it hard to love myself and to be nice to myself. I'm the first one to put my hand up and say that when things hit the fan, I'm the one to blame myself and beat myself up. That isn't such a loving action to do and you certainly wouldn't parent your children this way, would you?

We also must ask ourselves whether we give our power away or diminish it. When people give me compliments, I normally bat them away or say something silly. When I coached people with the Kick Ass Your Life principles, one of the things I told people is that if they don't receive compliments then they are not receiving the gift that it contains.

Receiving, I believe, is one of the hardest traits that a woman can embrace. We are always there for other people, nurturing and loving them, giving them gifts, but when it comes to us, we tend to forget about those nurturing and loving thoughts. In Chapter 1, we talked about harnessing our power, but we need to harness that power within ourselves and to ourselves, i.e. we need to become that loving and nurturing woman to ourselves first.

I used to hate that saying, 'love yourself first if you want to find a loving relationship.' This didn't mean much to me, but now I understand it more on a level of honouring, respecting, and, yes, loving yourself. I think it is one of the most difficult things to do in the self-development world. Even now I groan at that saying when I hear it. I wonder why. Is it a teaching that I need to hear repeatedly?

I know when I first got into self-development 20 years ago, I think I didn't even *like* myself. How could I love myself if I didn't even like me? As I've said, we are taught that our feminine power is wrong, manipulative, and over-emotional. How can we love that? We are not taught in school how to love ourselves, or even how to look after ourselves. I can't remember classes like that, can you? Even now, 20 years on, I am still struggling with loving myself, honouring myself, and respecting my 'warts and all.' It is a process. I think I do love myself now but do my actions clearly show that? I am not sure. Where are you on that journey?

Do you think it feels arrogant to say that we love ourselves? I feel we diminish our power so that others feel good about themselves. We don't shine because we are afraid that we might upset someone or overwhelm them with our shining. We cower in a corner until someone pays attention to us because we want to be needed and liked. Why don't we shine? Why are we afraid to shine?

What can you do to accept yourself as this amazing person? How can you use your feminine power to do good in the world and to yourself?

So, isn't it about time that we got into a relationship with ourselves? Bring our feminine power to us! How can we do that?

Sit quietly for a while and remember the things that you do to love yourself. Is it having a relaxing bath, taking yourself off for the weekend, or giving yourself permission to just chill out and watch a good film? Do you honour yourself by making choices that suit *you* and not to please others? Do you do what you love?

There will be things that you do already to love, honour, and respect yourself. Take a minute to reflect on what these are. However, be mindful if you are not living by them or forgetting what you need. Be mindful of how you treat yourself. What does it feel like or look like to have a relationship with yourself?

Relate to yourself first before you look at relating to others.

Relationships with Others

I asked this question above:

- In relationships, do you give your feminine power away or do you diminish it?

I know in my relationships with others, be that with family, my ex-husband, my mum and dad and sisters, I tend to lose myself or give away my feminine power. I have done this for many years. I know when I first had a boyfriend when I was 18 I hardly saw my family for six months. I totally fell into that relationship and to my detriment I lost myself. I tried to become someone I wasn't!

I have always felt that I need to be liked and accepted by others and feel this has been a common thread for all women who I have coached. Sometimes this feeling has led me to make decisions that were not in my highest power and detriment to myself for me to be liked.

Is that because we don't love ourselves or that we, as women, want to fit in as we like the idea of being in a community with others? We thrive around people, but I know for myself I totally become someone else, someone else that, I feel, other people would like. How bizarre is that? If I had already harnessed my feminine power, loved myself, and put my relationship with myself first, then I wouldn't do this. Would I?

After 25 years of marriage and 30 years of being with my ex-husband, I wonder if I was ever myself in that relationship. I know any relationship is all about give and take and sometimes we do things that we don't want to do, but when we broke up I did question whether I liked the walking we did, the places we went. I kept asking myself:

Do I actually like these?
Do I like these hobbies?
Are these places I wanted to go?
Are these hobbies what I wanted to do?

Do you feel like that in your relationships?

Take a moment to think of how your external relationships are serving you.

As I said before, you can also learn a lot about these relationships. I find when my friendships change or my relationships with my family change, it means that I have grown as a person, which is a good thing. Although losing these relationships seem scary at the time the ego voice might tell you that no other relationships are coming and that you have made a mistake to let them go. Don't fear. When I hear this voice, I must remind myself that these relationships that have fallen away or changed are because they were no longer serving me as a person and serving me right now in my growth.

Have you had a similar experience?

This is where you need to be courageous and loving towards yourself. When you reflect on the relationships you have with other people and find they are not serving you anymore, then maybe it is time to let it go! Make space for a new relationship to come into your life.

This may seem harsh as I write these words, it's not easy to let go of any relationships. I didn't let go of my 30-year relationship without working at it first and grieving that something I held dear to me ended. You will still go through all the emotions of ending relationships, either with a friend or a loved one. You will miss them, and you will feel sad, but on the other hand, it is time for you to put yourself first. Honour that this relationship is no longer serving you. You deserve more if you are unhappy in your relationship. It is time to love *yourself* more and deserve more in your life for *you*.

Sometimes we tend to repeat mistakes in our external relationships. I was separated for seven years, decided to have another relationship, and, lo and behold, found myself in the same patterns. It wasn't until I said to a friend, "This relationship reminds me of my last," that I decided to end it. I have grown enough to realise that I am worth more than just fitting into someone's life. I also must acknowledge that these are my patterns, which I also need to deal with.

These patterns that we tend to repeat in relationships are embedded in our conditioning. Sometimes we don't notice, but when we do it is like a déjà vu moment. I decided when I ended the last relationship that 'no matter how lonely I am, I deserve more'. I'm not going back into those old patterns.

Journal for a moment and think of the patterns that you might be experiencing in your external relationships. Are they serving you? Do you want more?

If you want to break free of these patterns then you need to come full circle, which comes back to your relationship with yourself. Yes, it does sound simple but this is where most of our pain is, the pain that we inflict on ourselves.

However, this is where the magic lies: the realisations and the learnings. Don't forget, at the beginning of this section, I said relationships are a great lesson and if you are single and are trying to find the right relationship, then read on.

Dating Again

If, like me, you find yourself single at this time of your life, it may be time to get out there in the world and seek a relationship with a partner. I know I miss that connection with someone. I have found myself dating in the twenty-first century, which is much different from when I dated at 19. It does sound scary but it is important to know what you value in yourself and others and what you can or cannot compromise on.

What I have found is that I am clearer on what I am looking for, but I need to pay attention to those red flags. I saw them on a couple of dates but I put up with them. I didn't listen and didn't put myself first. This is where it is important to harness your feminine power so that you can stand tall in your decisions. Knowing yourself better can lead to better relationships with others. By identifying your old relationship patterns and how they play out in your life can also be healing, if you are willing to change them.

When I first started dating again, my self-esteem and self-worth dramatically spiralled downwards. I found myself giving my power away. I had to harness my feminine power and become more self-aware. I had tears when some people blocked me after one date or never returned my texts. I was not clear on what I wanted so I would sound flaky to the other person.

Again, you may need to be clear on what you want and what type of relationship you are seeking. Getting clear at this stage will help you. I didn't, but maybe it is a steep learning curve. However, I believe the more you date, the more you become aware of what you want. I know I'm much clearer after being in the dating game for a couple of years on and off. My friend reminded me after yet another failed date that I was clearer on what I wanted and didn't want from a relationship. Every relationship or person you meet teaches you something.

Standing in your power will now be second nature to you but sometimes we waiver, especially when we are seeking love or a future partner. Remaining in your power is the key. Be confident in what you want and ask for it. If that person doesn't fit your desires or profile, walk away with your head held high. You might feel like that there is something wrong with you but don't forget do ask yourself whether *you* like them. I forgot to ask myself that, I asked whether *they* liked me and made my decisions around that.

Asking the latter question was me seeking approval from men, wanting them to say how beautiful I was or how attractive I was, but that doesn't work. Some men will also be frightened of powerful women who stand in their power, but again that is okay. You don't want men like that. They will find what they are looking for but it's not you.

Seeking External Approval

This is a common problem or trap that you might fall into. We all want approval from others, but maybe it is to dig deep and find out where this desire comes from. In my investigations, I found it was a conditioned part of myself coming from my childhood. I had to heal this part of myself to continue dating.

Seek approval only from yourself. As they say, love yourself first, but sometimes this isn't the problem and can be difficult. My advice would be to find the core issue of why you are seeking external approval. It might be your own beliefs, your own family situation or something that happened in your life. Get to the core of the problem.

Ask yourself: What do I gain from seeking approval from others?

Sit with this question, breathe into it, and wait for the answer from your intuition. Harness your power and see that warrior of a woman inside you. Ask from that place, not from the place of your wounded little girl, your emotional part. Click into your heart space, radiate the sun around your body, and ask the question.

Coming back full circle - YOU

After reading this chapter ask yourself these questions:

- Where do I need to change?
- Do I need to harness my feminine power?
- Do I need to love myself more?

These are important questions to ask yourself. If you think you have buried your feminine power and can't seem to access it, don't worry, you are waking up and connecting with more of your feminine power. Don't forget we have already established that you are a fab mother, you may have a fab career and a fab relationship so you must have feminine qualities to have all that magic in your life. When you connect more to your feminine power you will become aware of how amazing you are. You will be able to harness these qualities to allow magic to happen in your life (more on that later).

If you have identified what patterns you are running around relationships with yourself and others you will be able to heal these patterns to help you bring more magic into your life. You will be able to live a life more in your feminine power (that's the purpose of this book)!

Bringing awareness to what you think are your weaknesses, even if it's just a question of not seeing how great you are, is the key to transformation. I say this a lot in my first book, *Kick Ass Your Life*. Awareness brings change. Sometimes you don't need to figure it out, see a therapist, or spend years working it out. It is like an 'ah-ha' moment. See it, feel it, and then remove it.

It does sound simple and the concept is, but if, like me, you are more used to feeling bad about yourself and beating yourself up then you will lack this awareness. What we tend to do is, see it, feel it, and then hang on to it.

Is your pattern the same?

However, the magic is in the releasing. We don't even have to know what we need to release but by being willing to release what is no longer serving you will help.

I hang on to these patterns because I can beat myself up about it. I'm an overthinker and a psychic said to me recently I would be a good FBI agent. I need to ruminate on things, go over and over and over and over , and then, only then, when I'm on my knees, do I let it go. That sounds quite painful, but I'm being honest. Even though I've taught this stuff for years, it still gets me square on the nose.

Ask yourself these questions:

- What do these lessons mean?
- Am I willing to let them go?

What do I want?

This is a powerful question to ask yourself every day. By not understanding where you want to go to live a more fulfilled life, you will remain stuck in this circle of relationships. The only way out is to see more of your life, more of what *you* want to do. Be more in your feminine power to harness what you would like to see in your life.

You may not be able to answer that question yet but the next chapter will help understand your power and intuition. Asking yourself "What do I want" and listening to your intuition for the answer will be more powerful then listening to your ego mind.

CHAPTER 6

Law 3 - Understand Your Power and Intuition

"Understand your power and listen to your intuition."

IN THE LAST CHAPTER, we talked about understanding your relationships and, more importantly, the relationship that you have with yourself. Self-development is all about understanding who you are as a person, loving that person, and allowing yourself to listen to your wisdom to propel you into a more fulfilled life.

However, what we tend to do is to dismiss this power and our innate wisdom. We simply don't trust ourselves and our most important power: our intuition. Some might call it our 'gut instinct'. It doesn't matter, it is all the same. We all have intuition, but in women, I believe it is a stronger connection because of our feminine power. We can connect quite easily to it. That is why corporate jobs no longer serve women as it is too much in the masculine energy, which is to do, do, do. It's all about action, whereas feminine power is all about *being*.

Feminine power is sometimes about reflection and going with our gut instincts. Some of you may believe that this is coming from outside of us, this guidance, some call it spirituality, others say the Universe's ability to speak to them or simply they hear a voice but not sure where it is coming from. Whatever you believe the trust is that you have an ability to listen to your intuition which is an innate truth inside of *you*.

If we understand this power, then it makes everything easier. Our lives become uncomplicated and we literally go with the flow. We do not look outside of ourselves for answers and don't rely on friends to give us the answers. Instead we look inside of ourselves and follow our intuition.

Your Ego

On the way to following your heart and your intuition, there are some roadblocks to look out for. This is your ego talk, your ego mind which isn't part of your intuition and sometimes we don't know who is speaking to us. When I taught self-development, a lot of people asked me when they would know whether it was their ego or their intuition. I would say, "Your intuition is pure, pure love, whereas your ego is slightly bitter and self-justice." I know when I am in the ego mind as I tend to over-analyse things and feel angry and judgemental towards people. This isn't my intuition because it isn't pure love.

Just sit for a moment and see what your truth is. Remember a time when you just knew, deep down, that this was right, the thing that you were meant to do, you just knew! I'm sure you have had lots of moments when you just simply went with your gut. Sometimes these decisions are not logical, but you just knew it was right. That is your intuition. That is listening to your gut. Listening to your feminine power.

One of the things that happens to me is that I say to myself, I have lost my connection or I can't hear my intuition. That is mainly due to being stressed or tired. I get caught up in the *doing* and not *being.* When I am in that space, I tend to ask my friends what they think about the situation. Some of my close friends have cottoned on to this and they know to say, "I can't answer that," and "What do you feel?" These are the relationships that I want to keep.

Over the years I have concluded that I haven't lost my connection at all. I'm just not listening, or don't want to listen. Have you had an event when you felt it was wrong but did it anyway? It didn't work out, did it? I'm a stubborn person and tend to do this but on reflection, it was just a simple fact that I wasn't truly listening to my intuition. That is okay, the more you listen and act on your intuition the more your confidence in listening will grow.

Trust

In this ability to find your intuition and to listen to it, you need to learn to trust all aspects of this voice, this inner knowing. Maybe it comes through your body. You might feel sick when it's not right, or you just know. Sometimes this takes many years to finally trust in yourself, trust this inner knowing, and that is okay. We might make mistakes or take the wrong turn, but you need to trust that all is working out perfectly. Even though we find ourselves in a tricky situation or think of it as a failure. Listening to your intuition and inner knowing leads to trusting your inner voice. Therefore, the more you do what you feel and know, the more trust you will build.

This is all part of the trust process and might take practice.

Ask yourself these two questions:

- Have I had a situation where I didn't trust my intuition?
- Did I have a situation where I did trust my intuition?

Compare the feelings that you had. What did you learn and how can you take these learnings forward in your life?

As I said, we are all learning, improving, and growing, so don't beat yourself up. Hopefully, you will learn from these mistakes, but maybe you won't. I used to say in coaching sessions that if we don't listen, the Universe gives us a tap on the shoulder; if we persist then we get the sledgehammer. I now try to avoid the sledgehammer. But don't worry if you persistently get the sledgehammer, I've been doing this for over 20 years and still sometimes get the sledgehammer. It takes literally bashing me over the head or a slap in the face to get me to recognise that I am going down the wrong path. That is okay because the Universe always has your back.

Sometimes you might feel that you made the wrong mistake but still did it anyway. Don't worry because that mistake will also be a learning, a learning to trust your feelings and get out of the situation as soon as you can.

Trusting yourself takes practice, practice to listen to your inner being and not your ego. You have had lots of practice listening to your ego and therefore that is why it is so familiar. However, if you trust in your intuition you will notice a difference. It may come from a different part of your body or you might hear it differently. Trusting your inner voice and intuition can be unfamiliar, so practice, be gentle with yourself, slow down and find ways to help you to listen.

Ways in which we can listen

One way for me is to journal. I love writing and having been a coach for over 20 years, I love to ask questions. These are two of my superpowers. I sit quietly and journal and ask questions. If I receive an answer I write it down but it's okay if I don't get the answer straightaway. I make a conscious effort to write in my journal every day because this is a practice that helps me to connect.

The thing is, we are always connected but sometimes it feels like we have lost the connection. That isn't the truth, we have the connection. It's not lost, but, as I said before, we are simply not listening, that is the crux of it. Or maybe, you are not taking time to sit and just *be*. This is difficult and often we need to have a practice that suits us. It may not necessarily mean meditation, but something where you are *being* and not *doing*.

Below are some ways in which you can listen:

- Meditation
- Qi-Gong – a movement meditation
- Writing/journaling
- Being in nature
- Sitting in silence

- Yoga
- Chanting
- Sound healing
- 5 Rhythms Dancing

Add anything else that you find helps you. Make a list so that when you are feeling disconnected you can see from your list what you need to do. Sometimes when we our too much in our ego mind we forget what helps us to connect to our intuition. Our ego wants us to avoid that activity because it doesn't want us to connect. When we connect the ego mind is not in control which it doesn't like.

Having read some of Eckhart Tolle's book about being in the present moment is helping me. I didn't understand it for a while but I went to a mindfulness workshop and could really see the benefits. If, like me, you have an overactive mind, and overthink a lot, this is a challenge, but one worth the attention and practice.

When you are in the moment, everything is working out, you have no money worries, you have food on the table, and a loving family. When we look to the future, that is when our ego mind will go crazy. We cannot predict the future, so we need to just keep stepping forward and taking the next step, whatever that means for you.

Remember: trust takes practice. Practice and you will find yourself always listening to your intuition, your inner knowing.

Harness your words

As I have mentioned above, it's important to be kind to ourselves. Listening to our intuition and understanding our power takes time. When we listen and act on our intuition trust is then built. Therefore, along the way we must learn to harness our words.

The Mother Elders remind us:

Be good to yourself and others. Sometimes you will procrastinate and beat yourself up. This cannot be accepted in the feminine power. If you have this power, then how would you treat yourself? To return to Law 1 about harnessing your power you must really understand this power and investigate it yourself. This can only be done from a positive outlook. When you are tired and stressed you are oblivious to all good things. Try and stay in a positive state no matter what and watch out for the words that you speak about yourself and what you say to others. Harness your words to all the greater good.

If we understand our power, then we must remember that our words create our reality. Therefore, we need to be careful in what we say and think. I know when I am stressed and tired I am very good at beating myself up, and this is how I lose my connection with my intuition. My ego takes over and does a really good job. How about you?

Connecting and developing your intuition comes from a place of positivity. By understanding where your ego tries to take you is a power within itself.

Go back to Chapter 1 and try to understand how to harness your power and then harness your words. The Mother Elders remind us that these are both important so that we can listen to our intuition, to make choices from our feminine power and not our ego mind.

When we remain in our feminine power and connection then it is easier to stay in effortless flow.

CHAPTER 7

Law 4 - Remain in Effortless Flow

"Seek approval only from yourself."

THE MOTHER ELDERS REMIND us that to remain in effortless flow we must stay within our feminine power and seek approval only from ourselves. We are divine beings and our inner wisdom is the truth. Therefore, we do not need to seek approval from outside of ourselves. As I said in my second book, '*The Authentic You*', when we seek approval from outside of ourselves, it leaves us feeling overwhelmed and confused. The answers are all within us and that is why we must connect with our feminine power.

We tend to give away our power when we are in relationships and seek approval from others. I have found myself doing this when I have been back in the dating game. Seeking approval from men. Why do you think that is?

People would say to me that I am beautiful, amazing, clever, and successful, but I don't see any of this. I am blind to these compliments as I don't believe them myself. Do you find yourself in those patterns too?

People can tell me that I'm wonderful many times, but if I am blind to these qualities then they will fall flat. I simply won't believe them. They are just words which don't mean anything to me. So how can we validate ourselves? What does this mean?

Validation

Validation is something that we tend to seek from outside of ourselves rather than validating ourselves.

Sit and journal and ask yourself these questions and think of a time when you have done this:

- Do I ask friends what their opinion is before making a decision?

- Do I ask friends/family whether I am a good person?

If you have answered yes to the above, then you are seeking validation from outside of yourself. When you have harnessed your feminine power, seeking approval from yourself will become easier.

However, the patterns of seeking approval from others will keep playing out. This is coming from your conditioned self and not your feminine power. Awareness is key to try and catch these thoughts and patterns. These patterns are not coming from your feminine power, they are coming from your ego mind. This takes practice so try writing down where and when you have done this and how you felt. This will help you to transform this part so you can be in effortless flow and more in your feminine power.

You can also seek validation from your relationships. If you have been in a relationship for many years and you are now single, then it is likely that you miss someone telling you that they love you and to compliment you on how you look. When was the last time that you told yourself that? Probably never. But why do we do this? It is just our conditioning. Have you ever heard the phrase, 'put others first before yourself'? That it might be selfish to think of yourself. However when you hear the safety announcement on an airplane, they will tell you to put your oxygen mask on first, and then you can help others. An interesting thought?

Women tend to meet other people's needs before we meet our own needs. I know I've done this when bringing up my children. I'm running a family home and looking after the children I was the last person to think of. It then becomes a habit of not nurturing ourselves when we are feeling tried. We only stop when others people's needs are met.

You might find this pattern more prevalent when your children have left home. We stop and don't have the distractions that this home life brings. When we have this space, this void within us that we are trying to fill with distraction. We have simply lost the ability to know what we want to do and how we need to nurture our bodies. We are used to looking after others.

I tend to keep busy all the time because then I won't need to listen to my inner being and my ego mind is in control. I can then run on empty and treat my body badly, eat badly, and don't recognise what harm I am doing. What if your body and mind were your best friends? How would you treat your body and mind then?

When I taught self-development, I always used to say, "Only say things that you can say to your best friend." This automatically stopped people in their tracks. If you spoke to your best friend in the way that you speak to yourself, what would you say? Journal the thoughts that are currently in your head.

What would your best friend say about those words?

It's an eye-opener, isn't it? That is something to ponder on.

Ask yourself:
- When was the last time you validated yourself?

Seeking approval from others seems like the easy route to take, but what if they said that you were a horrible person and that you complained all the time? Would you believe them? I know for many years living with my ex-husband I believed those things and didn't have a voice. I believed their words because I believed them myself. What an irony!

How do we validate ourselves?

To validate ourselves you must honour yourself. Honour your opinions. Honour your successes. Honour your voice.

Having a voice

It is not all about shouting from the rooftops, "I am amazing!" (why not!) but it is speaking up and honouring what you want. How many times when your kids were growing up did you do things you didn't want to do? Yes, sometimes it is all about compromise, but other times we need to say NO. But when was the last time you did something totally selfishly for yourself?

When I teach people how to write a book, the voice is one of the most important aspects to master because people want to hear your opinion, they want to hear your story. So, the voice must shine through without doubt.

Journal and ponder this question:

- When it comes to my life do I have a voice?

  o If yes, what does it sound like?
  o If no, what would that voice sound like?

I know when my kids left home and I felt all alone, my voice sounded harsh and pushy. Sometimes my inner voice said punishing words of, "I'm not good enough," and "I am a failure." When we say negative things to ourselves our bodies react. We become ill, or our back gives way. Again, it is going back to beating ourselves up.

How does your body react when you say negative things? Do you even notice?

Having been a practitioner of Kinesiology for many years, I know that the muscles can do two things: be strong or be weak. When I test negative things on clients then their arm goes weak straightaway. How powerful is our body? So, when you say negative words and eat unhealthy foods, you are walking around with weak muscles.

Does that scream feminine power to you? Are you harnessing your feminine power or taking it away?

That's a good thought to have, isn't it? What if you didn't hear my voice in this book? Would you want to read on, be interested, or put the book down?

These are all things to consider and don't forget that I am going through this process with you as we walk forward together into a new chapter of our lives. I do these things. I am not a guru, but I am my own guru. I have noticed these things within myself and, as they say, you always teach what you have been through. I have done that in my other two books, too. I have kick-arsed my life and tried to live an authentic life. Now I am having to learn about my feminine power.

Have a powerful voice

What if you had a powerful voice? Not only for yourself but around others. Would your friendships and relationships change? Would you be more successful? This is something that I am pondering too.

What if I validated myself and had a strong voice? I wrote a long list of positive things that I would be and do if I validated myself, nothing negative, so why are we dimming our voices and our lives?

As I said before, a lot of this conditioning is because we are women. The world is slowly changing, but we still have a whole load of history that tells us that women are the weakest sex. In some parts of the world, women are still classed as second-class citizens. We believe this conditioning; it is in our DNA. It is only when we awaken to our behaviour that we begin to question what our lives would be like if we had a voice and harnessed our feminine power.

Isn't it about time that women are more powerful? And it starts with you. You can't change anything in the world unless you change yourself.

As Gandhi said, "The western world will be saved by a western woman." How powerful is that!

Shine a light on your power

When I taught a lot of clients how to change their lives, I advised them that they needed to shine a light on their behaviour and how they treated themselves. By doing this it brings self-awareness and you begin to see the patterns that you are running and therefore you can transform them.

Without this awareness, you are blinded by your power, by your beauty, and by your amazingness. You are also blinded by what you need to change and what you need to make better.

However, sometimes it is painful to look inside of ourselves, to be willing to see our imperfections or to see our patterns of how we see ourselves. It amazed me one time when I was treating a Kinesiology client. She was scarred to open up. She said, "what if you find something that is horrible." I then explained that the fear is coming from her conditioned self, the one who she sees as imperfect and maybe a bad person.

I have this ability when I do healing, to look inside the soul of a person. The very core of who they are. What I see is only beauty and love coming from that core. I wonder how many people think that they are bad to the core. That is not your feminine power, it is your conditioned self.

By shining a light on your power rather than the negative or conditioned part of yourself, how would you see yourself?

Journal the answers to these questions:

- What do I see or feel when I look inside my soul/the core of my being?
- What would it feel like if I only saw beauty?

Shine a light on your power and believe that you are amazing.

If you are struggling to see who you are, then this meditation will walk you through to shine a light on your soul. Are you ready?

Meditation - Shine a light on your Soul

Find a quiet space so that you are not disturbed.

Place your feet firmly on the floor and close your eyes if you wish.

Breathe in.

Breathe out.

Take a moment to appreciate the surroundings that you are in.

Enjoy the quietness or the sounds that are around you at this moment.

Take a deep breath and release.

When you are ready, surround yourself with pure white light.

Breathe in this light and know that you are protected. That anything that you see is coming from your highest good and not from your ego mind.

If you have any negative thoughts then this is coming from your ego. Just let these flow past without any judgement and surround yourself with more white light.

The white light is coming from outside of yourself, beaming down on you, shining a light on your feminine power. Bask in this glory and know that the Mother Elders see you in this light.

Breathe in.

Breathe out.

Take a moment to connect to the sun shining in your heart, you can radiate this sun around your body whenever you need to. This is your feminine power.

Make the sun brighter and brighter. Surround your whole body in this light.

When the sun becomes brighter it reveals your soul, the beauty that is inside of you. The pure essence of who you are.

Don't be scared and don't fear this power. Your soul is pure beauty, it cannot be anything else.

Just take a look into your soul. What can you see?

Are you kind? Caring? Thoughtful? You might see or hear some words or you might see some colours. Feel anything that you are feeling come to you naturally.

What colour is your soul? Is it pure white, the colour of the sun, or something else?

Take a moment to connect to this image and get to know yourself intimately. Smile and your soul will smile with you.

Keep connecting to this pure essence of yourself for a minute or so.

When you are ready, allow this image to just be. Wriggle your fingers and toes and come back to the present moment.

Immediately after you have done this meditation, please journal your feelings, thoughts, and anything that you saw or felt. Every time you do this meditation you might get a different image or feelings and that is okay. Try not to judge whatever comes. If you have difficulty connecting to this power, to your soul, then connect to the feeling that you got when you did this meditation. You can call upon this feeling anytime you want to stand in your feminine power.

When you have shone a light on your feminine power and know who you truly are, you are ready to learn more about your purpose and whether this needs to change for the new chapter in your life.

CHAPTER 8

Law 5 - Find Purpose in Life

"Purpose on this earth is just to be you".

IN THIS NEW CHAPTER of your life, you may be seeking another purpose in your life. You may feel that you have lost your identity or purpose now you are not a full time mum. You may feel tired or have little or no energy in what you do and that is okay.

When we are in perimenopause we are letting go of old things, bringing forth the new and this may include you questioning whether you are in the right job or just want to do something new.

Maybe you are feeling depressed or lethargic because you have no direction in your life and feel you are just drifting. You feel that there is something else out there that you want to do. An adventure. That is okay, you are in the right place. In this chapter, we will look at this aspect of your life to give you a new direction, a new purpose in life. You will feel renewed and passionate about your life. Hold on to your seats, you may be blown away.

How are you feeling right now?

Let's sit with this question for a minute. Tune into your feminine power and ask from that place. Remember, take your emotions out of the picture for a while and see if you can connect to that wise woman that we found in previous chapters. If you need to, revisit the meditation where you met this wise woman and then ask these questions. Journal your answers:

- Do I feel I am on track?
- Do I feel there is something more?
- Where are these feelings coming from in my body?

When we feel like there is something more that we need to be doing, we have this ache inside of ourselves, generally around the solar plexus area which is just above the belly button. We just know we are not on track and know there is something more. That is okay to be feeling like this. Sometimes we try and deny it, saying that we are fine and lucky. You may find yourself in a fortunate place and grateful but that doesn't mean that you don't want more. Especially at this time of your life where you are finding yourself with more time, more *me* time that you are unsure of what to do with it.

I don't like wasting time. I like to feel productive with my time, but sometimes I go over the top and go into burnout. What I forget is that this downtime is important to listen to my intuition. When I am not receiving messages, this is because I am too busy. I don't sit and just be. I know when I am not because I journal every day. When I look at my journal it has one page when I don't connect and when I do connect there is a difference in the writing, it has several pages of my thoughts and not just what I have done. I also note that when I'm feeling the most vulnerable and emotional the pages are blank. This is when I need to connect more but I don't. That is interesting, isn't it? Do you find a pattern in your journalling or writing?

When I allow myself to sit quietly, I can hear my wise woman shine through. I can hear her voice and her wisdom. When I don't allow myself this time, when I am too busy with *things*, I shut this voice out and feel like I have disconnected. Sometimes we don't want to hear, we are fearful, or just don't have the headspace to listen, but you must find some time. Even if you don't hear your wise woman, or you sit and meditate with no information or no answers, it is still worth it to sit still and be mindful of your body.

It's not logical

When we do listen to our wise woman don't be surprised if you hear something that isn't logical. I did. When I asked about my next step after my children left home, I received a message to travel through Europe. And so I did. This was a challenging journey, but a trip of a lifetime which I enjoyed thoroughly. But it wasn't logical. I sold everything, moved to London, 150 miles from Bristol and my family, and then into France and Italy. This didn't make sense to me because one of my main values is family, so to move away from them all was alien to me and frightening, but I acknowledged what my wise woman was telling me and went for it.

It wasn't easy. When we change direction people think that it is a bed of roses, but in order to change there is always fear and pain which we need to push through. As Susan

Jeffers always said, "Feel the fear and do it anyway."

It's not easy

Let's look at this: it's not easy. You may see other women just going for it, moving away, getting a new career, or entering a new phase in their lives. You may see them and think to yourself, 'It looks easy, she did it. Why does it feel hard for me?'

Let me tell you something: they would have gone through the pain and fear just like you. When I told my friend that I sold everything and travelled, she said, "You always just go for it. You make it look easy." I told her that it wasn't easy, I had to go through a lot of doubt, mostly doubting myself and my abilities, and a whole chunk of fear! With the help of my friends, I had to overcome those feelings, and just did it anyway. Therefore, it may look easy on the outside but it isn't.

Therefore, I feel it is important when people say, it's easy, it's important here to tell them the truth, to be open and honest that you are finding it difficult. It's okay that it's not easy. I always think that if it was easy then every Tom, Dick, and Harry would be changing their lives. They are not. You are because you are reading this book, trying to grow and to move forward.

Well done, you. You are one of the few who will dive deep into their thoughts and feelings to grow.

Get clear on the next step

Sometimes we don't need to know how the rest of our lives will look, even five years from now, as it is too big a jump into the future. I think of the next step only and when I was travelling around Europe, I found myself living in the moment, in the now, and I had no fear, no worry, and went with the flow.

I see many people get stuck and never grow and change their lives because they are overwhelmed by the question of: 'What do I want?' As I said above, this is a loaded question and you will feel overwhelmed by the enormity of trying to sort out the rest of your life.

Therefore, break it down into sections. If it feels right to just ask your wise woman for the next week, next month, or next year then that is okay. Feel what is right for you. If you are a planner you might want to plan further in advance. Making a plan is all well and good but be careful that it is not too rigid. Going with the flow and making changes when it is needed is the key here.

When travelling, I met other people who were travelling and I asked them about their biggest challenge as a traveller. They all said that they must be adaptable and change when it is needed. They might plan something, their flight may be cancelled or their hotel is not available but they pivot, they adapt to whatever is going on. That is sage advice for any new traveller, but also a traveller through life.

Being rigid will not allow the flow, of new things coming to you, new opportunities that you might miss because you are being too rigid. I wasn't planning to go to Verona, but having met a traveller who was born in Verona I decided to go. It was the best place I visited because it wasn't planned. I went on a whim, and I loved it. I allowed myself to go with the flow and embrace the change, the detour that this provided me with. I sat round the pool, looking out at the sunset over the vineyards, which I would have missed had I not taken the Verona guy's advice to go and visit. If I had been rigid and said, "It's not on my plan of places to go," then I would have missed this opportunity to see a beautiful place.

Allow yourself to flow

Coming back to perimenopause and menopause, the flow of menstruating is stopping or has stopped, and you might also be feeling this in your life and body. I find myself in perimenopause sometimes thinking that my flow feels stuck, and I get frustrated. The flow of the body is that it doesn't have to bleed every month but does still get emotional and tired and that is okay. It's a different kind of flow that I get to embrace. Are you frustrated with where you are in your life? Is your body slowing down?

Are you getting cross with yourself because you aren't where you think you are supposed to be in your life, that you have no direction? Maybe you don't need to know what the next five years will bring. But being super clear on the next few weeks will allow you to embrace the flow more easily. Embrace that flow, embrace knowing what your wise woman is telling you. Stand in your feminine power, don't deny that power, that flow. Embrace it and allow it to be.

Emotions are like the flow of life, the flow of your body. Some days you may feel like crying or happiness may be an overriding factor, embrace that and allow that to flow. Don't judge but allow it to be. Sometimes we criticise ourselves and beat ourselves up that we are sad but if you accept that this is part of you, part of your inner wisdom and your feminine power you will back in the flow. Again, harnessing your words is so important to allow the flow of your life. Thinking '*I am in the right place at the right time*' allows you to release the pressure and allows more flow into your life.

How to live a more fulfilling life

This is a question that came up for me when I spent three months in Italy. I was unhappy with my life; my business wasn't doing so well and I lacked motivation and passion. When I journalled, I was asking myself the question, "What do I want?"

That question seemed huge and I didn't know how to answer it. I kept going round and round in a circle. Nothing was coming from my intuition. My wise woman was silent.

When I became aware and listened to my intuition, I began to ask another question that I felt was a more empowering question. That question was, "What does the next stage of my life look like?"

When I asked that question, I felt a lightness inside of me. It triggered an excitement inside of me and I began to get some answers.

You may want to sit down and ask yourself the first question that I asked:

- What do I want?

Reflect and journal what your intuition is telling you. How does your body respond?

Become aware of how your energy is. Are you struggling? Does it feel too big of a question to answer?

Then ask yourself the second question:

- What does the next stage of my life look like?

Reflect and journal what reaction you are having to this question. Are you more excited? Does it feel like the right question?

Notice what your reaction is because the first question might be the right one, but for me, the second question felt so much lighter. I got excited and the answers flowed.

Consider this, maybe you are asking yourself the wrong questions in other aspects of your life. What we don't realise is that sometimes we may be asking the wrong questions. We simply beat ourselves up and give up, saying, "I can't do this, it's hard." But when you ask the right question, a more empowering question, it begins to fill you up with excitement. It is about asking the 'right question' for you.

When I asked the right question, the more empowered question, within minutes I had my list. This is what I received:

- ✓ A loving relationship
- ✓ A beautiful home
- ✓ Stable income
- ✓ A chance to grow
- ✓ Freedom
- ✓ A job or work that I love
- ✓ Friends
- ✓ Loving relationships with my children
- ✓ An active social life
- ✓ A tribe
- ✓ A new spiritual connection with myself and others
- ✓ Travel to see new places and meet new people

I was struggling for weeks with, "What do I want?" but when I asked a more empowering question, the answers began to flow. I don't know how I'm going to achieve them, and they might change, but in that moment, I had answers that I didn't have before. I, therefore, began to trust my intuition, my feminine power that I did have the answers that I had been searching for.

It shocked me a little that I wanted a beautiful home. I gave up my home after my children left home to travel and I didn't think I wanted a home. Maybe I was in the wrong business, or I needed to make changes in that business to be fulfilled.

I had friendships but maybe I needed more.

I had loving relationships with my children but maybe I needed to increase that.

There are some aspects that I already had in my life and maybe I just needed to increase that contact or that connection. Sometimes we don't need to reinvent our whole life, we don't need to start building something new. It may be the case that we need to build on what we have already. It is easier to build on the foundations of what we already have rather than to rebuild. Change is not always about something new.

You never know until you start uncovering how you want to be fulfilled. This may seem a little daunting but don't worry because you cannot start living a fulfilled life until you start uncovering the answers.

I asked the Mother Elders why we don't seem fulfilled and this is what they said:

You seem unfulfilled when things need changing or when you are not recognising what you have already. Look around and be grateful for the things you have. However, feeling unfulfilled is a sign that you want more or that you want to grow more spiritually. Spiritual growth will allow you to bring more into your life and that is what this feeling could be. It is not about being unfulfilled with the life you have now but that you can bring more into your life. That is the ultimate question. When we experience spiritual growth, we expand into more of who we are, and that involves having space for more in our lives. It is also a choice to let go of dead wood in your life: people, things, or behaviours that are no longer serving you. Being unfulfilled is something not to be feared but to be celebrated as you step into your power, stepping into your feminine power. Therefore, celebrate it with your friends, sit around a campfire, and talk about these things. Don't fear that you want more. It means that you have simply grown into your power. Celebrate.

Wherever you are in your life right now is the perfect place to be. Be aware of the things that you already have and be grateful. Sometimes we don't necessarily see what we already have in our lives. Begin a gratitude journal, being grateful for whatever is in your life right now. Be grateful to the growth that you are experiencing, the new learnings and relationships that are coming into your life. Be grateful for everything because you will then start to see the beauty in your life already which will help you stay more in your feminine power.

If you are struggling with your purpose, then tune into your feminine power with this meditation.

Meditation - Finding your Purpose

Find a quiet space so that you are not disturbed. Place your feet firmly on the floor and close your eyes if you wish.

Breathe in.

Breathe out.

Breathe out all your negativity and things that you are holding onto.

Breathe in.

Breathe out.

In your mind's eye see yourself standing on top of a mountain. You are looking down on a beautiful landscape. You can see grass, a beautiful big tree, and colourful flowers. This view makes you feel calm and relaxed.

As you take in this view you see yourself down there amongst the flowers, leaning against the tree. You are detached from this person but you know that this is you. You have similar qualities and you just know that this is yourself, your higher self, this calm self who holds all the wisdom.

Breathe in.

Breathe out.

This person sees you looking down at them and looks up to meet your eyes. You wave and say hello. This person invites you down into the landscape. "Come on down."

You float down and feel yourself beside this other person, you sit facing each other within the beautiful flowers with the tree beside you both. The tree provides the support you need to really look at the other person.

"What wisdom do you have for me today?" you ask this other person.

"I have loads of wisdom for you. What do you need to know?" she replies with a smile. She touches your hand, and you feel reassured.

"I've lost my way. I don't know what my purpose is," you answer her.

She looks into your eyes and you feel a sense of security, a sense of knowing that you already know the answer.

"All you need to do to find your purpose is to look within. Embrace me as your other side," she says.

You may feel a little uncomfortable, but you know deep down that this is the right thing to do.

You are blinded by a white light that is coming down from the sky and you look up. Momentarily blinking, you need to know where the bright light is coming from. As the bright light dims, you blink and look towards the other person. You may panic a little because you can't see her clearly. You feel frustrated that she didn't answer your question about purpose but you remember what she said.

"Embrace me as your other side."

You close your eyes and you feel something merge within you. You feel this bright light coming from your heart and you clearly see this other person, the person that you viewed from on top of the hill. The inner wisdom, you.

You connect with this person. You embrace this white light and place your hand on your heart.

And say, "Thank you."

The question is no longer relevant as you know deep down that you hold all the answers. Whatever your purpose is, it will be okay. You can decide what that is.

You then ask, "What do I want my purpose to be?"

You feel more empowered than waiting for an answer to "What is my purpose?" You can decide what your purpose is. This is okay as it can change, but you have an inner knowing that it will soon be revealed to you and that you will feel at peace once more. There is no need to worry or to push anything. You can just relax and wait for the answer to be revealed.

Give thanks to the realisation that all the answers you are seeking are within, it is not coming from outside of yourself and you can decide. You can feel what is right and what is wrong. You can decide for yourself what your purpose is.

You feel excited now that there is a choice and not something that an outer source is telling you. You feel rejuvenated to go and do different things, go and find different groups of people, or just be you. You can discover what your purpose is by how you feel.

Sit for a moment to feel this excitement course through your body. Give it a colour and move that colour around your body. Let it be for a minute or two.

Don't force the answer but it may come, you might feel it, you might hear a word, you might see a picture and you might not. That is okay. Wherever you are in the moment is okay. You are in the right place at the right time.

Breathe in this colour. Breathe out this colour.

Breathe in this feeling. Breathe out this feeling.

When you are ready, let go of this image, wriggle your fingers and toes, and come back to the present moment.

This meditation is powerful because you switch the question around from 'what is my purpose?' to 'what do I want my purpose to be?' We all have a choice, but I think we forget this as we lean more into our spiritual practices. We feel that we must wait for the sign, for that feeling to *tell* us what we need to know but we are in charge. It is our feminine power that we tune into, not something outside of ourselves. It is coming from our feminine power within ourselves and this meditation will help you to tune into that power.

Be more in your feminine power and you will find that asking a different question will help you get the answers more quickly. You will feel more empowered and less dependent on what others say. You are the sign, you are the decision maker, and no one else is coming to save you, to tell you what to do. Be reliant on your feminine power, your inner wisdom and knowing. This is how to live a more fulfilled life and harness your feminine power.

Now that you might have some direction around your purpose, it's time to look more closely at how to develop your inner knowing and trust the signs and direction that you have been given.

CHAPTER 9

Law 6 - Develop Your Spirituality

"Spirituality is a practice, a muscle that you build up every day."

THROUGHOUT THIS BOOK YOU have been developing your spirituality by tuning into your feminine power with the meditations.

How do you feel after the meditations?

Do you feel stronger?

Do you feel you are more reliant on your inner wisdom?

As the Mother Elders said in Chapter 8, when we feel unfulfilled, we are ready to grow more spiritually. Maybe the transition from perimenopause to menopause is our rite of passage into leading a more spiritual life. Therefore, feeling unfulfilled means that we need to be spiritually open. It is interesting that in my list of 'what does the next stage of my life look like' I listed, "a new spiritual connection with myself and others."

How interesting is that?

I had a dialogue with the Mother Elders about spirituality and why we seem to see this as a thing that we do to ask questions when we are in trouble. Why this isn't part of our routine?

When you tap into this spirituality you will live a more fulfilling life and find your power within. No one else has the answers. They are all within us. I find myself too easily asking trusted friends what they think instead of enjoying the quietness so that I can listen to my spiritual side. It isn't freaky or woo-woo. It is always there but something we don't tap into. The theme throughout the previous chapters has been how to harness your feminine power, how to listen to your intuition and build your trust in it.

I had a lot of questions about this subject which I asked the Mother Elders. This is what they had to say about this.

Q: Mother Elders, how do we develop our spirituality, so we feel at home? How do we stop the ego from wanting more, more from others, more from things? How can we be comfortable with ourselves and with our feminine power? Why are we frightened of our spirituality and our power? Why can't we shine?

A: *Being with yourself is not easy. We remind Ann of the time when she did some healing work and her clients would be fearful of when she tapped into their systems they thought she might find something wrong, that they didn't like but in fact what Ann saw was the beauty of their soul, no matter what they did, it was still beautiful and colourful. What women fail to see is this beauty. They harness their power on what went wrong, what they did wrong, and only see their faults. This is where returning home and returning to your spiritual side will enable you to let go of all these hurts, these feelings, and misdemeanours. You will only focus on the beautiful side of you.*

This is difficult because all your life you have been taught to fit in. You don't want to outshine people and be different. I bet most of you have wanted to fit in and were very different at school and with your family. That is something to be celebrated, not feared, not diminished. You chose to be here on this earth to be different, to not fit in, and life has brought you many lessons of this, ones that you perhaps haven't yet learned.

You are all being called to come home to yourself. This is difficult because you were never taught this. We as Mother Elders have not been diminished. In our culture men have always seen the beauty of women and their power and we have remained strong in our community.

To find yours, connect with spirit or your higher self, because when you do, everything is good, you feel happier, you don't need others, you don't need things. However, this connection may feel alien because you have been taught to please others, to be with others and this doesn't allow your spiritual side to develop. It is diminished, and you will find yourself being someone you don't like.

Whatever spirituality is to you, it may be meditation, it may be just watching a good film, or it may be just spending time alone or with like-minded people. No matter what you do externally you will always find your spirituality inside.

Q: How do we find our spiritual side?

A: *You don't need to find anything. It is always there. You have just lost your way of accessing it.*

To access it you need to be quiet, to pause, and to consider what the messages you receive mean to you. You need to be in a healthy place. That doesn't mean you need to heal your past, that is not relevant, but you will see the signs if you connect with your spirituality. Don't let life sweep you along. Be mindful and consider your own inner knowing.

Ann, you have done this but denied your connection. This connection that you are having with us, the Mother Elders, you have doubted and denied the voices in your heart all along. You have developed spiritually because you are now beginning to listen, but you lose the connection and that is why we are here guiding you. You always had this ability as a child, and you spent time alone, but people made it wrong. However, having a deeper connection with yourself is more important than looking for that connection through other people.

Connection with people is important too, they teach us a lot, but if you have spent time as a child in this spiritual realm then you wouldn't be frightened. If you tap into your ego, it will tell you that you are lonely and don't have any friends, but if you tap into your spiritual side and your inner knowing it becomes easier. You know everything is working out perfectly, you don't have to be or do anything, you are content.

Ah, breathe in this relief that everything is just perfect. Give gratitude for this. The search is over, you have come home to yourself.

Q: Why is it frightening to be at home with yourself?

A: *It is not frightening; it is just unfamiliar. We haven't been taught to sit with ourselves, we have been taught to ignore our feelings and keep going. Get used to the unfamiliar, to connecting in this way. When you do, you will find more people who are doing this, being with themselves, although you don't need anyone at any moment in time. Things are working out perfectly.*

When you have this calling, it is time to be on your own to fully understand this concept. Don't get busy with relationships, either men or women, quiet your ego mind and just be. Do the things that you want to do, write, and expand your mind without any limitations. It is a freeing experience. You are safe, you are loved. That is all that matters. The Universe is bringing you everything you want in divine perfect timing. Lighten up, it is only fear that will keep you stuck.

Enjoy the beauty of within. Enjoy your life and whatever lessons it is bringing you. Show your creativity through writing, drawing, or painting. Get back to the quiet within. Back to your beauty and your feminine power.

Get rid of all the distractions in your life and just be.

What an interesting conversation that the Mother Elders have given us. It is unfamiliar to connect with a higher power or whatever you want to call it. It is familiar to listen to our ego mind and our fears. I am always reminded of this when I travel and visit new places because I am in the moment. I am seeing new things and it doesn't remind me of where I have been or my past. It is simply new and exciting, and I can be myself, and be in the present moment.

I think that is why I tend to write more when I'm travelling because I allow myself the time to just be, with no pressures of work or family. I have no responsibilities; I can simply be *me*. I tell my friends and family that I am travelling for three months, and they seem to leave me alone. They respect that I am away and allow me to be me.

For years I haven't been allowed to be me. We all conform to what others expect from us, what a responsible mother and a person of my age look and act like. When I'm travelling, I seem to be youthful. I don't have a fear about what others think because I don't know anyone.

They don't know me, and they don't have any expectations.

Maybe this is the question that you might like to take some time to answer. Journal your answers. Ask yourself:

- What does it feel like to be me?

Maybe we have forgotten to ask ourselves this question. Maybe we have lost touch with ourselves and with our spiritual side. Don't forget that spirituality isn't separate. We don't lose connection with it; we simply don't listen. Or life and our fears take over and we don't remember that we have something stronger inside of us other than our ego.

Connecting with our power and spirituality is all one. As the Mother Elders have reminded us, we haven't lost that connection, it is always there. It can be loud or sometimes a whisper. However, it is still there. I can hear my inner connection more powerful when I am quiet and calm. When I'm stressed it feels like I've lost the connection as it is a mere whisper.

What stops us from building this spiritual connection?

The ego mind can stop the flow and will prevent us from doing those things that will bring us joy, that will bring us closer to our connection with our spirituality. When I write books I get out of my own and drop into my heart and the words flow.

Like the Mother Elders remind us, spirituality is just a practice that we can develop over the years. It may be yoga, it may be journalling or writing, or taking 10 minutes a day to meditate. This brings us closer to our spirituality, to our connection to our source. When I was in Bali I did Ecstatic Dancing, which in essence is an inner dance, dancing from your intuition and allowing your body to freely dance. This allows the head space to be quiet. I enjoyed this as part of my spiritual practice and it's something that I do now regularly. There are always new ways to connect to our spirituality. However, some things bring us further away from who we are, from our spirituality, and to that connection.

Procrastination

Procrastination brings us further away from who we are, and from our connection and fully embodying what we want in life. It stops the flow which disconnects us from our inner knowing. Be mindful of when procrastination takes over your life. You may begin to feel stuck and unable to move forward. If you are feeling frustrated and overwhelmed then you may be procrastinating.

Have you ever felt like that before?

When we are aware of procrastination and when it shows up, we can begin to create a spiritual practice that we can stick to. The more we connect the more we feel alive and present, and the more we are likely to do something.

As the Mother Elders reminds us, this practice is like a muscle that you build up over time. I know meditation doesn't work for my connection. I would rather be active, so my meditation is my inner dancing or walking meditation that allows me to connect and let my head be free of any thoughts. Running also gives me this quietness in my head.

Don't make any practices wrong that allow you this space to grow and truly listen to what is going on in your life. Everyone is different and some people can meditate and sit quietly and others cannot. Find the right thing for you. The more we connect, the more answers we hear, and our lives will become easier in the process.

When we stop and allow the quietness in our spiritual practice then we are more at peace with ourselves.

No more working it out! No more controlling your every thought and feeling. Let it be, stay present, and allow your spiritual practice to take over.

What do you feel is your spiritual practice?

We have talked about listening to our spiritual side, that inner powerful voice, but how do we simply reconnect with it when we feel our connection is broken? What do we need to do?

As mentioned above, we may find our spiritual connection by doing activities such as:

- Walking
- Meditating
- Walking Meditation
- Participating in Qi-Gong
- Yoga
- Being in nature
- Connecting with like-minded people
- Journalling
- Writing
- Being creative
- Dancing

There is a whole list of things that you can do but you need to find something that fits you, fits your personality, and how you like to connect. Or simply ask your feminine power what she needs.

Write in your journal the things that you currently do to tap into your spirituality. Then add a few more new ones that you would like to try.

I connect through my journal, being outside in nature, being by the sea, walking, and in the last year, I have been practicing Qi-Gong, which is very beneficial in allowing me to see the wood from the trees and to release stuck emotions.

This spiritual practice connects you back to your feminine power. Some people may feel that they can't connect because they need to heal their past. They are not in the right space to allow that connection. But let me tell you that you are in the right place, you don't need to heal your past or be on a different spiritual path. You just need to connect with your inner power, to you, that is all there is. You are in the right space, at the right time. Everything is working out perfectly for you.

How we see ourselves stops us from trusting and fully immersing in our feminine power and our spiritual side. Drop the illusion and give yourself permission to be you.

CHAPTER 10

Law 7 - Drop the Illusion

"Drop the illusion - see who you are with a new set of eyes."

THE MOTHER ELDERS REMIND us that we must see our worth and drop the illusion of who we *think* we are. Who we think we are is just a conditioned mindset that we are holding on to. It can be seen as a veil hiding the real you. However, the real you is much more powerful.

When we step into our feminine power and drop the ego, this is where magic happens, where our lives become more fulfilled and exciting.

Who are you?

Have you heard yourself say, "Who am I?" Do you seek guidance outside of yourself? I know I do. I visit psychic therapists and ask my friends for approval. Is that because I am unsure of who I am? Or is it something else?

At the time of writing this book, I had a hard time seeing my worth. I became aware of how others were treating me, including myself, and feel now that that is not okay. That is not how I want to treat myself anymore. I've realised that if I don't treat myself with kindness and see my worth, then how can I expect others to treat me that way too? Suddenly, I felt free of everyone's expectations, particularly my ex-husband, and now can I truly be me. Free of all limitations that others put on me and what I put on myself.

The Mother Elders have advised that we must see ourselves with a new set of eyes from our feminine power, from a place of love and acceptance. It is time to see yourself.

When I received this message, I didn't think much of it, but now that I can see my worth, it makes so much sense. The word 'see' is very prominent in this sentence. See yourself in the mirror. See who you are. This is interesting because it is not saying, "Let others see you, let others decide your worth." As we all know, self-development and change are inside jobs, but if we externally see others treating us badly, or our career isn't going so well, it is easy to drop into 'I must not be worthy' or the classic saying or belief is 'I'm not good enough.' Have you heard that limited belief many times in your head?

I know this has played out in my life and have fallen into a trap of when others can't see my worth then they must be right. Don't forget, how others see you may not be a reflection of who you are but a reflection of what their beliefs are and how they are projecting them onto you.

When I got into the spiritual world, I hated when therapists and coaches said that you are a reflection in the world, i.e. if you hate yourself then you will experience that externally but sometimes that didn't seem true to me. I have been trying to disprove this theory for years!

I think that maybe if we feel bad about ourselves then we simply attract that. We manifest that idea of who we are but not necessarily the truth. What we think about ourselves is untrue or just an illusion.

A lot of people find the alternative/spiritual world when they are stuck. I know I have and still do. In my first book, *Kick Ass Your Life*, I thought of self-development as uncovering the beauty of a person. There is nothing to fix. What self-development is doing is bringing awareness to your conditioned self and of what *you think* you are and uncovering the beauty that you have forgotten. It's not about becoming a new person; it is about uncovering the real you.

It's my fault

I've always had this belief that 'it's my fault.' I must have said something wrong and not done enough. My friend did some NLP (Neuro-Linguistic Programming) with me on this belief and afterward I started challenging people about what they were saying. My son came round my flat and I opened the door that went out onto a small balcony. My granddaughter was sitting on my lap and we were looking out of the door. My son came along and shouted, "Mum, watch Rosie, she might fall out."

I looked at him strangely and my ego fully took hold and I thought that he didn't think I was responsible enough, that I would allow my granddaughter to fall out of the door. Instead of this thought, I challenged him and said, "Why would you think I would allow her to fall out?

She couldn't anyway." He then explained that as he was a new parent, he was overprotective of his daughter (as a new partner will be) and he had fears about her hurting herself. See, a simple explanation. It wasn't about me at all, he didn't think that I couldn't care for her and allow her to injure herself. It was his own fears about being a new parent.

In recent years I would have gone down the rabbit hole of thinking over and over again that I was an unworthy nanny and that I had done something wrong. But by simply questioning him, I uncovered a lot about him and his thinking, not about me at all. It brought a softness to the moment, without blame and anger, and I saw my son for the loving parent that he is.

This belief may stem from our childhood but this is something that you don't have to believe. You can simply unlearn it. However, you must be aware of it first. Awareness is key and transformation can then begin.

Next time a person is horrible to you, just imagine that it wasn't about you but what limitations the other person has or how they see themselves; how they are seeing themselves in the mirror and how they are projecting that onto you. If you know the person well, see back in their past and if they were treated badly or had a terrible experience. Now can you understand why that person is the way they are? Most of the time it is not about you at all.

Who am I?

I think this is the question that most therapists and psychic people are asked! I know when I was a coach and therapist, this question came up time and time again. I know I have been searching for this answer myself. It is interesting to note that the Mother Elders advise us that there is no path to finding yourself and it's a mystery to human beings. I suppose we go back to my argument that "you don't need fixing." But this can go deeper. So, let's break it down. If we don't need to know 'who am I' there is no path to finding yourself, what is self-development all about? Why do people seek externally for the answers that there is no answer to? An interesting thought.

If there is no path to finding yourself then what are we seeking? What is the real question that we are asking internally and externally?

Maybe it is, "Am I okay with who I am?" "Am I enough?" Is it approval that we are seeking from others? We know who we are and what our purpose is but is what we are seeking from others what we cannot give to ourselves?

Another interesting thought. What do you think? What is coming into your intuition?

Take a moment to journal your thoughts and add anything else that you may find challenging.

The Mother Elders also say that what you *think* about yourself is untrue, so what are we listening to? Ego? Are we driven by our ego mind and not our true self, our heart? It is also interesting that they say that they have eyes in their hearts and that is why they can see beauty in us, only the positive side to us. We all have different sides to us. If someone pushes my buttons enough, I will snap and get angry, but that doesn't make me an angry person. I'm only human.

When I was a therapist, people would come in and say, "I am depressed," or, "I had a bad day and got angry so, therefore, I am an angry person." Of course, that is not true. They are not an angry person, and neither are they a depressed person if they are sad. That is a sweeping statement and one that can be damaging as it might become your identity. The 'I am' statements are particularly powerful as you are labelling yourself.

Perhaps the Mother Elders are right in that we are not seeing the real person. We are just seeing the limited version of ourselves, the one that we have been told we are.

If we drop that illusion, the illusion of who we are that we have carried for many years, perhaps we will begin to see the real person. See who we are and realise that there is no path to finding ourselves! In fact, we have been here all the time. Now that is a thought!

See yourself

If we drop the illusion of who we *think* we are and see through the eyes of love, through the eyes of our hearts, and not of our mind, what do you see? I know when I coached people, I only saw their beauty. There was no judgement. I could see the beauty in everyone that came to me.

Wow, I had forgotten that. Why don't I see myself through those eyes with no judgement?

What are your thoughts? If you saw through the eyes in your heart and not through your ego head, what would you see?

Ponder that question for a moment as this is a powerful statement. It allows us to not *think* but to *feel*. Do you feel that you are an amazing person? Or do you still feel that you don't know who you are?

Fundamentally, you know what type of person you are. I know I am kind and caring deep down and that is the essence of me. I can feel that I am kind, but my ego mind would then try and take me down the rabbit hole and say, "Well think about that time yesterday when you got angry and judgemental at work for one second." After that thought I could believe I am not kind and caring.

That makes total sense, doesn't it?

Drop the illusion

With that in mind, you know who you are and you know what you are seeking. Everything else is just an illusion, something that the ego mind keeps telling you. If you dropped the illusion, what would you see? Close your eyes and let's see if we can uncover the beauty of you.

Try this meditation to help you:

Meditation - Uncovering the Real You

Find a place where you can be quiet and undisturbed. Take a few deep breaths in and out. I invite you to close your eyes if you wish.

Breathe in.

Breathe out.

Breathe into your feet, breathe into your legs, breathe into your stomach, into your chest, and your neck. Let go of all tension.

Take a deep breath in.

Breathe out and release everything that you are holding onto.

Connect with your solar plexus, the space just above your belly button. Connect with your feminine power. Radiate the sun around that area.

Breathe in.

Breathe out.

In your mind's eye see a picture of yourself as you are. What do you see?

Connect to your inner voice. What message has it for you today?

Take a few moments to really connect and listen.

Bring awareness whatever your experience, there is no judgement.

Breathe in.

Breathe out.

Connect back to your feminine power and come from a place of strength. Radiate the yellow of the sun around your body.

You can now hear the feminine voice. That powerful one that has strength and can see who you truly are.

Breathe in, breathe out, and let go of any tears that may form.

Don't regret anything, you are here now. You are in this space so be thankful that you are letting go of anything that may come up.

Bring the colour yellow into your solar plexus and radiate this colour all around your body. Shine the beauty within. Feel the warmth of this colour.

What do you see now?

Do you see the strong woman that you are?

Can you see your strengths more clearly than your weaknesses?

Breathe in.

Breathe out.

Celebrate this woman. Cheer her on rather than putting her down.

In your mind's eye visualise yourself inside a circle of other women. They are surrounding you and you are dancing around, arms outstretched. You are taking energy from these women. You are celebrating. They are clapping, they are cheering you on. They see you. I see you. They see the beauty within, they smile at you as you take on their positive energy. They see you. Do you see you? Do you see this beauty within you?

Stretch your arms out to your side and dance around. You are this brilliant woman, who has been through a lot, and who is now in a new chapter of her life. This is you.

Shout out, "This is me!" Keep dancing.

Be supported by the women in the circle. This is your tribe. These are the women that will celebrate you and keep you on track when you are feeling low. Take this energy and place it within your heart, within your solar plexus.

This is the essence of you. Take a moment to soak this feeling in.

Breathe in.

Breathe out.

When you are ready let go of this image, wriggle your fingers and toes, and come back to the present moment.

What illusion did you have to drop? What veil were you wearing? Take time to journal your thoughts and the visions that you saw. These might change over time so it is good to keep a record. You can see how far you have come.

It's time to see yourself

No one is coming to save you! I've had this thought many times throughout my life. When I spoke to a large audience, I felt that I needed to have confidence within myself that it was coming from me, not externally - no one was coming to save me. I needed to reassure myself.

When you shine your light, everyone can see which can feel scary. What is stopping you from shining your light? What is stopping you from seeing yourself?

In the above meditation, women are celebrating you and not tearing you down.

That's why it is important to find your tribe which I talk more about in Chapter 10 – being part of a community.

I hope the above meditation helped you to see yourself and to help you drop the illusion. As you practice this, it will get stronger and stronger, and you be able to stand in your strength in the truth of you.

If you are struggling a little and still saying to yourself, "Is it worth it?" then let me ask you this:

- If you don't see yourself in this new light, where is your life heading?

When I ask myself this question, it is a scary thought that I might be stuck here where I am now and unable to move. It's time to stand up, put on your big girl pants, and stand in your feminine power. It is beautiful, you are beautiful, and it's time to drop the illusion and see yourself with your heart. Drop the illusion of the ego mind and start believing that you are an amazing and powerful woman.

CHAPTER 11

The Unspoken Law

You are the Mother Elder!

AS I AM WRITING this last chapter, I have come to realise that I am not channelling the Mother Elder, nor is it coming from the Universe. It is coming from my feminine power, my inner wisdom. Before, I believed that the Mother Elders were external but in fact they are my inner wisdom, they are a part of me.

I am the Mother Elder!

How powerful a statement is that?

The Mother Elders remind us:

"See yourself sitting around the fire being the Mother Elder. You are wise. You have a wealth of wisdom. See yourself as that powerful woman with a purpose. You have returned to yourself, to your higher power, to your feminine power."

Your Mother Elder is a returning to yourself, returning to your home, your feminine power. I am so excited to have been able to recognise this within me as I write this book, and I hope that when you have reached this chapter you are also excited to be returning to yourself, to your inner wisdom, to your feminine power within *you*!

I was reminded of this when my friend did some NLP work on me to help me stand in my power. After that session, I meditated and tried to bring in my Mother Elders to ask for their assistance as I have done throughout this book. When I first envisaged them I saw them as wise women who were giving me advice and I would always sit on the end. However, this time I was invited to sit alongside the Mother Elders and they were asking for my advice also. I had indeed became one of them. I had returned to my rightful place alongside the Mother Elders.

This is an interesting concept to consider. If all my wisdom or the Mother Elders were within me, why haven't I used them for my higher good? As the Mother Elders remind us:

"We have forgotten to access this part of ourselves. We only access a small part of our feminine power."

How do you feel being a Mother Elder? Does this excite you? Does it frighten you?

This book started with finding your feminine power, but as I've reached this part in the book, I am reminded that this is not the ultimate goal. Being a Mother Elder is.

Throughout this book, you have learned how to harness your feminine power and how to use your feminine power positively so that you can grow to become a Mother Elder. To recognise that Mother Elder within yourself.

We all have wisdom to share and when we harness our feminine power, we become one of those wise women who sit in a community. That is why a community is important as stated in Chapter 10. Don't forget these Mother Elders do not sit alone, they are sitting with other Mother Elders sharing their wisdom.

If you haven't got to that point of becoming a Mother Elder, don't worry. We all grow at difference paces. Don't forget you are in the right place at the right time.

This visualisation will help you get into that state, to truly believe that you are a Mother Elder. You may feel it already as you move throughout this book, or you may need to go back and revisit some of the chapters. In any event, you are a Mother Elder because you would not be reading this book and you wouldn't have read this far. This book would not have resonated with you.

Meditation - I am a Mother Elder

Find a place where you can be quiet and undisturbed. Take a few deep breaths in and out. I invite you to close your eyes if you wish.

Take a deep breath in and out.

In your mind's eye, you see yourself standing tall, standing in your feminine power, proud to be you, free of judgement.

You are open to all possibilities.

In your mind's eye conjure up a picture of the Mother Elders sitting around the fire. The eldest

Mother Elder invites you in and you walk into their inner circle.

The Mother Elders are sitting on logs and you look around at their faces and nod.

You envisage yourself standing tall and in your power. You feel strong. You feel confident. You belong with these Mother Elders.

As you do, you see a space open up. The Mother Elders invite you to sit down.

You sit down and you feel at home. This is the place that you have been searching for. You feel safe. You feel secure. You feel like you belong. You are a Mother Elder. Breathe in this feeling.

The other Mother Elders pat you on the back, they welcome you and say, "Where have you been? We have been waiting for you to come and sit with us."

You are not scared anymore of owning your power, of standing in your feminine power and you feel a positive energy around you.

The fire is blazing away in the middle and a Mother Elder asks you, "Have you any wisdom for us today?"

You take a deep breath and say, "Yes I do."

You see all the other Mother Elders stop talking and they all look at you. They are waiting for your wisdom.

You take a deep breath and say whatever comes into your intuition.

You feel safe sharing this knowledge. Maybe something is going on in your life but you feel powerful, you are being heard and your feminine power, your yellow light that shines within, is shining brightly. You have a powerful voice.

You ask the Mother Elders, "What wisdom have you for me today?"

They reply, "Only be yourself, stand in your feminine power. You have all the wisdom you need. We are only here to guide you, to make a safe space for you so that you can hear your intuition loud and clear. Do not be afraid of what comes to you. Follow your intuition and be true to yourself. Start this next chapter of your life with vigour, have fun, and be playful, everything is working out perfectly."

You thank them for reminding you that your intuition is strong and that you are indeed a wise Mother Elder.

You sit for a while in the presence of the Mother Elders without the need to speak. You just take in their energy and feel their loving presence.

Take a deep breath in and out.

Harness that feeling of belonging, the feeling of being a Mother Elder.

Take a deep breath in and out.

When you are ready let go of this image, wriggle your fingers and toes and come back to the present moment.

This visualisation reminds us of our return to our feminine power. A return to being a Mother Elder. And that what we harness inside of us, is true wisdom. Our wisdom. Nobody else's. We are all unique and we are indeed part of a wider universe than we realise.

We are not alone. We can tap into these Mother Elders and sit with them when we feel lonely and when we haven't yet found or built a community of others. My wish is that there are more Mother Elders rising and as we stand in our feminine power the more women we will find around the world that will have created communities.

CHAPTER 12

How to Rise Collectively as Women

COMMUNITY IS GOING TO be important in the coming years. When I speak to the Mother Elders I envisage them sitting in a circle around a fire, speaking their truths and sharing what they have discovered.

This is something that we have lost in the western world but something, I feel, that is going to be important in our lives once again. We need to *get into* community, especially women. We see this at the school gates, and in nurseries, but we do not see this so often when our children are grown up. When we are at this stage in our lives we feel alone.

We have wisdom to share with others, and powerful teachings that, like the Mother Elders, we can impart with each other and the next generation. When we are in community, we are more powerful, we feel supported and therefore we enrich each other's lives.

You may feel that you don't belong anywhere now that you have reached this stage in your life, but we must find ways to feel that sense of coming together. We may perceive that we have been bad mothers, bad wives, or not used our femininity in a way that we now understand, but all these snippets of information, good or bad, help other people.

All our experiences count. It is whether we view them as bad or good that stops us from sharing them with others. My bad experiences may help others not make the same mistake and my good experiences might inspire others that they too can achieve it.

As I said at the beginning, COVID has separated us from our loved ones and mental health is more important than ever. That is why community is so important, to feel part of something. It doesn't have to be our family, but how would you feel if you sat in community with other women in your same situation?

- Would you feel lonely or separate?
- Would you feel included and heard?

The choice is ours and we have learned in the *7 Laws of Feminine Power* that women and mothers are powerful. We have a wealth of information that needs to be shared.

Loneliness

When we sit in community and have that connection we don't feel lonely. Since the children have left, I have felt loneliness and loss as I transition into a Mother Elder and continue the next chapter of my life. This is the definition of loneliness from the Oxford Dictionary:

> *sadness because one has no friends or company; feelings of depression and loneliness; the state of being alone and feeling sad about it*

However, I don't believe loneliness is a lack of friends as you can feel lonely when you are out and about with friends. I believe loneliness is a lack of connection to the right people. I know now that I need deeper connections with people, otherwise I will become bored and unsatisfied.

You can also feel lonely in company - do you? You can feel lonely in your relationship - have you? Therefore, loneliness cannot be a definition of not having any friends or being alone.

I travelled last year for three months and realised that I do like my own company. Living in a co-living space with others I felt that sometimes I wanted to be alone, to do my own thing, and to just be me. If I am around a lot of people all the time I feel exhausted and want to recharge. I am an empath and so this is the way that I am. Therefore, loneliness cannot be 'the state of being alone.'

Do you feel lonely?

At what times have you felt lonely?

Where were you and what were you doing?

Test the theory above and see if it resonates with you. I have many friends and my family, and sometimes I still feel lonely. I can feel lonely sitting in a restaurant with many other people, living in the same house as my friend, it is simply not a lack of company, but loneliness is a lack of *connection*.

As I have said, it must be the right connection. As we evolve more into being a Mother Elder, we will be seeking out those relationships that fulfill us, that excite us, and which we feel part of. It is no longer relevant how many close friends you have. I only have a couple of close friends and that is okay. I have lots of acquaintances and know a lot of people, but I am choosing whom I welcome into my inner circle.

Community

That is why community is important. It is not a coincidence that I envision the Mother Elders as a group of women around the fire. It is not one Mother Elder that I communicate with, it is a community of them sharing their wisdom. They are a collective, sitting with each other in community.

The Mother Elders are calling us to build communities in which we feel a part of and held, to create communities to nourish our souls so loneliness is not a part of our western life.

What can you do?

You can start by using your feminine power and tapping into your higher self to ask yourself this question:

- What can I do to create or join a community that will serve me and others?
- Are they like-minded people?
- Do they add something to my life?
- Do I feel safe and secure to be me within that community?

Community is important so you can be vulnerable, you can say what is going on with you, and be truthful about if you are having a rough day. It's not all about feeling happy. You can also share your wisdom about menopause and the effect that it is having on you without judgement. You feel that you can be open and share anything with this group.

On the other hand, we must practice not having judgement towards other people. This can be hard because we are hardwired to judge other people, to compare ourselves against them. Is she better than me? Am I good enough? Watch when these negative patterns appear and just sit with them. Feel no judgement. You have evolved into a Mother Elder and therefore your wisdom is important.

Honour and love yourself as a wise woman, a Mother Elder.

CHAPTER 13

The Mother Elder

MY HOPE FOR YOU is that you have become the Mother Elder as you reach this conclusion, but if not, don't worry, there is still plenty of time. Go back and revisit some of the chapters that you have found challenging. Everybody moves at their own pace. Perhaps you haven't been listening to your intuition or perhaps you have heard it but don't yet trust it.

As with everything it is a process, but you can use the visualisation in Chapter 10 as many times as you want to connect to the Mother Elders to help with this process. This will help you trust your intuition more and create a relationship with your higher self. Or you may want to visit the chapter on how to connect to your higher self or how to harness your feminine power.

Let me reassure you that wherever you are in this process, it is exactly where you need to be. You may need to learn more things about yourself, about what you want and that is fine. Don't beat yourself up about where you 'ought' to be or where you 'should' be. Simply just let it be and let the process take shape.

I found writing this book very therapeutic and it has helped me in my quest to begin a new life without my children, to begin a new chapter. Rather than looking at it as being scary, I see it as exciting and having fun. No pressure, just taking one day at a time.

As I have been writing this book I have been travelling again and this chapter was written in Italy where I am reminded that I mustn't compare myself with others and that I can go with the flow. Everything that is happening to me, perceived as good or bad, is the right thing for me.

The Mother Elders' wisdom came to me in the part of my life where I most needed it and I hope you have felt the same. This book has been written from the heart and not my head. I haven't figured it all out, but I have experienced all the chapters that I have written about. It has truly been a lesson for me also.

I write from my heart to your heart in the hope that this wisdom will help you transition into the wise woman that you are, to be present in your feminine power, and to be the Mother Elder. This is the ultimate goal to reach as a woman in transition.

About the Author

ANN LAMB STARTED HER journey in self-development by being a holistic therapist practising kinesiology, aromatherapy, massage, and reflexology. She has helped hundreds of people to change their lives and saved a woman's life in her career.

Ann then transitioned into a Life and Business Coach helping more people have a better life and business. She saved a client from losing £1 million in her business by helping her realise what she wanted in life. She has been teaching self-development for over 20 years.

She now has an international publishing business, Forward Thinking Publishing. They publish mainly non-fiction books but have a fiction arm. All the books that she publishes add to people's lives to help them nourish their souls. She once said to her friend, "My dream job is to read books all day." That dream has simply come true.

She has written two other self-development books, *Kick Ass Your Life* and *The Authentic You* under her married name, Ann Hobbs. Ann is also in the process of writing two fiction comedy novels about her travels around the world.

She is a keen traveller and her love affair with Italy continues. She has three grown-up boys and two granddaughters.

Be careful because if you do meet her on her travels, you might well indeed become a character in her book!

Where to find Ann

Website: www.forwardthinkingpublishing.com
Facebook: www.facebook.com/callannhobbs
Instagram:
www.instagram.com/forward_thinking_publishing

Find her books on Amazon under Ann Hobbs:

Kick Ass Your Life
The Authentic You

Acknowledgments

Thank you, dear reader, I hope it has helped you to grow and that reading this book has nourished your soul.

To the Mother Elders for trusting me with this information.

To Sam Cross for helping me getting this book into shape. She could clearly identify the difference from when I was writing from my heart and when I was writing from my head. Hopefully, I've rectified those places where my ego mind slipped in! I felt reassured and honoured that she recognised that this book was written from my heart.

To my clients who I have seen over the years, you have been an immense help in my development as a writer and a person.

Especially to three of my clients that have now left this earth.

To my children, Chris, Nick and Harry for the inspiration that they give me every day.

www.ingramcontent.com/pod-product-compliance
Lightning Source LLC
Chambersburg PA
CBHW071712020426
42333CB00017B/2229